You set your limits!

A Shockingly Useful Book

Everything Is in Your Hands

Emiliya Belcheva

A life-changing book!

A Shockingly Useful Book

Everything Is in Your Hands

Emiliya Belcheva

BOOKS

London, UK
Washington, DC, USA

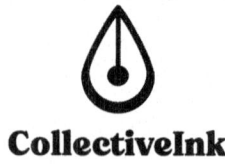

CollectiveInk

First published by O-Books, 2025
O-Books is an imprint of Collective Ink Ltd.,
Unit 11, Shepperton House, 89 Shepperton Road, London, N1 3DF
office@collectiveinkbooks.com
www.collectiveinkbooks.com
www.o-books.com

For distributor details and how to order please visit the 'Ordering' section on our website.

ISBN: 978 1 80341 644 1
978 1 80341 696 0 (ebook)
Library of Congress Control Number: 2023948054

Design: Lapiz Digital Services

UK: Printed and bound by 4edge Limited
Printed in North America by CPI GPS partners

The pieces of advice in this book have been carefully estimated and checked by the author. However, they do not replace competent medical statements. This is why the information in the book is provided without any guarantee by the author. No responsibility for personal, material, and property damages shall be sought by the author and her proxies.

Shockingly Useful Book
A life-changing book
First edition

We operate a distinctive and ethical publishing philosophy in all areas of our business, from our global network of authors to production and worldwide distribution.

I dedicate this book to all people who want to be healthy.
To all of those whose beauty does not wash out with water!
To those like me who are planning to live until 120 at least!
To my husband who is always there for me and has been supporting me for more than 15 years!
To my children who motivate me to make the world a better place!
To my parents who gave me life!
And to you!
Because life without you makes no sense!

Love,
Emiliya

Welcome, Fairy!

When I am lecturing – I am Emiliya Belcheva. I am known for my trainings for dropping the metabolic age, extending life, tissue and organ regeneration, losing weight, preparing diets, post-partum recovery, strengthening the posture, healing varicose veins, acne treatment, tightening the facial contour and removing dark circles, wrinkles, double chin and many more related to health. I am founder of Belchevi Health Academy, SEMMA (a sport treating backbone curvature and asthma), the only for the moment representative of "Академия Красоти ЮЛИИ Сайфуллиной" – Moscow. An author, lecturer and most of all – a mother of two.

I don't plan on bothering you with my personal story. If you want to know it – go to our website – semma.bg. There you will find various topics and materials that I used to change the life of many people. As at this moment, with the republishing of *Shockingly Useful Book* I have a total of three books. And let me give you a tip: I have a surprise waiting for you at the end of this book!

You don't need to do a thousand weird, time-wasting things to be in shape. It's all very simple. Stop harming your body and it will regenerate itself. In 2019 I am 31 years old and yet my metabolic age is 14. This is the age of your tissues and organs. And it has nothing to do with actual time. **You can't steal a twenty-fifth hour in a day for yourself but you can steal a year, two, three... ten. If you know how!**

This is why I wrote this book!

To teach you how to change your routine habits so you can be healthy. The things you still do every day, 365 days in a year define you. And this is what you least pay attention to. Why? Turn them from something mundane into something useful that helps you. Save time, be more with your family or yourself. Don't lose this!

As a mother of two, a housewife, workaholic, career-obsessed and a woman with many injuries from my birth, I had to choose. The family or me. I combined them! These pages will show you how you can do it too! Now people stop me on the street to take a photo with me because I changed their life with a free video or an article. The feeling is unique! To be useful and to know that you help! I want to help you too!

Don't neglect yourself! You are the most important one! If something happens to you, what will they do then? Take care of yourself, Fairy! Magic is not inexhaustible, you need to know how to recharge it. **Don't wait for the cup of emotions to overflow, nor for your strength to run out. There is no better day than today!**

My mission is to prolong people's lives and change the world together. Are you ready for a different point of view?

Feeling good is amazing! You owe it to yourself!

I used to say: "I hope things change."
Then I found out there is only one way to change
everything – change myself.

Jim Ron

Size Doesn't Matter: Carrots and Leaves

I want it. I will get it.

Henry Ford

When I was pregnant for the first time 6 years ago, I met the team of Jamie Oliver in Bulgaria. Parents and children could go cook with them and learn new things about how healthy vegetables are.

I was amazed!

And I learned something I have been using for 6 years now!

You eat carrots, right? And do you know how to choose them? Big, small... color... what about the leaves – what do you do with them?

Does size matter? – Absolutely **"Yes."**

Here I see a lot of men smiling **"I told you so!"** In the core of the carrot are the saturated sugars. There is a saying – "The bigger, the sweeter." Which means – more calories! But more energy as well! Smaller ones have less sugars.

What did I learn? The leaves!!! It's a magical ingredient which I had been throwing out for 24 years! I saw how they washed it and put it in the salad. I was shocked! **Carrot leaves** are a valuable source of iron, phosphorus, calcium, cobalt, zinc, boron, sulfur, sodium, nickel, copper, manganese, iodine, silicon. They also contain vitamins C, B2 and folic acid.

Potassium lowers blood pressure and is an ingredient in osteoporosis products. The ingredients in greens help **the kidneys to function. Vitamins A and E** are the most powerful antioxidants. They cleanse the body, something like a cold shower after power training. We release toxins from the body, slow down the aging process. We enhance regeneration and metabolism. **Vitamin K and chlorophyll** (which is not present in the root) help purify the blood and adrenal glands.

4

Nowadays, the pharmaceutical and cosmetic industries are spewing thousands of detox pills. All products are based on vitamin A, E, chlorophyll and the like. Vitamins are not chemically produced! They are extracted from fruits and vegetables, put in small tablets and sold to us! Why? Because it's easier to take a pill and you're done. Are you really done? These tablets also have stabilizers, they have one useful ingredient and 10 more harmful ones.

All this is stimulated by our way of life! We're always in a hurry... nonstop in a hurry. There is no time! We've become the "Alice in Wonderland" Rabbit, the one with the watch who keeps saying he's late. Instead of being calm, walking slowly, finding his gloves, taking everything and arriving on time, he was just jumping and constantly repeating there is no time. We all have the same time! We are all going to the same place! The question is how to get there! To cheat the system and steal more time!

Let's go back to the carrots.

In life all happens suddenly.

Andre Moroa

Chlorophyll, vitamin A, vitamin E – antioxidants. Do not wait to feel sick, saturated with toxins and heavy metals, but constantly cleanse your body. As you take a shower every day, so take these ingredients daily too!

Parsley and the green part of carrots have diuretic properties. Regular use prevents the appearance of kidney stones and aids breakdown of existing ones.

How to choose nice carrots? In addition to a strong orange color, they must have hard, fresh and green small petals!

Fiber helps the digestive tract. The colon is cleared, the abdomen is lowered, there is no swelling and pain. There is no feeling like a "pregnant cockroach"! Cellulose helps us maintain a slim figure, helps to lose weight and, as already mentioned – frees the body from harmful toxins. And **falcarinol** strengthens the colon.

Carrot leaves are very useful for diabetics, as they suffer from vitamin A deficiency.

Carrots differ from other vegetables with their increased content of potassium salts, which are vital for problems with the heart, kidneys and blood vessels.

Carrot leaves are rich in minerals such as potassium, calcium and vitamins A and B. All these substances strengthen bones and prevent osteoporosis.

Dream as if you will live forever. Live as if you will die today.

James Dean

Doctors regularly recommend eating carrots if you have eyesight problem. But the green part itself is more suitable for the purpose. Vitamin A is good for the eye muscle. In addition, beta-carotene is a powerful antioxidant that helps protect against muscle degeneration and the development of senile cataracts – a leading cause of blindness in old age.

And did you know that the real, first carrot was purple? Yes! It is artificially made orange, as a form of revolt in France. In this way, people supported the then successor, whose color was orange. And so, they both supported the ruler they wanted, not their current one, and they did not lose their heads.

Antioxidant properties are very effective in dispersing the accumulated mucus in the ears, nose and throat, sputum in the chest and helps with sinusitis.

The chefs told me that wonderful day: "The greens of root vegetables are many times more useful than the root itself. It is in the sun. It is saturated and nourishes the root." Many people think the opposite. BUT it is mutual. The root nourishes the leaves and the leaves the root!

This is true not just about carrots.

The successful person is always an incredible painter of their imagination. Imagination is more important than knowledge because knowledge is limited – imagination is infinite.

Albert Einstein

How to store them?

Keep away from apples, pears, potatoes and other fruit and vegetables that produce ethylene gas. They make carrots bitter.

How to grow carrot greens?

Cut the carrot at about 2 cm before the top. Put in an appropriate pot. Add water to cover about half a centimeter of them. Place near window. If necessary, add water. In about a week you will have your own fresh leaves. Another option is to put them in a plant pot with soil. Very soon you will have fresh leaves.

Eat fresh!

Live a full life!

Live a happy life!

The choice is yours!

Never underestimate yourself. You can do everything others do.

Brian Tracy

Salt

Great minds set goals; the rest follow their wishes.
Washington Irving

How to choose the right one?

Why do we feel like eating salty foods? – because we have a deficiency of minerals in the body. Do you remember back in the village how grandparents gave goats and sheep a big piece of sea salt? The animals made small dips in it from licking. I didn't understand why then.

What does salt actually do in our body and why do we need it?

I will allow myself to quote a paragraph from the textbook written by my brother – Kristiyan Belchev.

Removes excess acidity from cells and especially from the brain – helps balance the blood sugar – it is needed for the absorption of nutrients through the intestinal system. And as you know, most of them are absorbed there. Helps against muscle cramps – it is needed for a healthy bone structure.

Refined salt – often contains an aluminum anti-caking agent (it causes toxicity), as well as other ingredients that lead to water retention, high blood pressure, kidney problems, etc.

Unfortunately, refined salt is everywhere! Olives, cheese and everything salty has this kind of salt, unless it is explicitly written on the label – "with unrefined coarse sea salt." Most often it causes the limbs to swell, you get a severe headache. One of the reasons for this is the processing of this salt in order to extract the minerals from it and then sell them in the form of tablets and supplements. Top of the top was after I read a post on this topic two years ago. It described how cat and dog food are the only foods for which all over the world they have to prove that they can sustain life for a year, provided that the animals eat only this. The idea is really shocking. We need the minerals to exist in the right way. How to get it? Pills!

If you give up on your dreams, what will you have left?
Jim Kerry

How does the brain work?

It releases a substance that makes us feel like eating salty foods. We start thinking about olives, cheese, chips, popcorn and what not with salt. Once in our mouths, the stomach releases the enzymes needed to process food and extract minerals. The salt reaches the stomach and... there are no minerals! The brain repeats the action again and makes us eat salty food once more. If, so far, we have needed 10 units, then we already need these 10 plus 10 more (which had to process the second enzymes). So, in the end we constantly want to eat salt in every meal. I am often told in consultation: "I do not eat salty." In fact, we eat salt in the form of cheese, sausages, olives, etc. Our legs and arms are swollen. We cannot concentrate. Our fingers are swollen every morning, we have bags under our eyes, cellulite, etc. I really like to give Pepi as an example, she listened to me and replaced only salt in her diet thus losing 2 kg plus all the swelling in 10 days.

We process the salt with chemicals, extract the minerals and put them in animal feed and in supplements. People buy salt to have a salty taste and will buy more and more because they need it because of the deficit. Finally, they switch to supplements.

Either you manage your day or your day manages you.
Jim Ron

And the answer is very easy! Eat salt!

But any kind of salt?!? Himalayan?

NO! It is a stone standing in the sun, with a salty taste – earth salt. It is not alive! We will talk about the negative charge soon! Its charge is positive! It is dead and has a salty taste. You can eat some cardboard with the same effect.

"Earth and refined salt have an altered molecular structure, they remain in our body for a long time, swell joints and cause kidney problems.

"Unrefined sea salt – 78% sodium chloride, 11% magnesium chloride, less magnesium and potassium carbonate and traces of other important minerals." – again, quoted from Kiko's textbook.

Imagine how sea salt is formed – in the sea! Minerals are grouped together by the evaporation of water and accumulate. It is alive. We don't feel like eating even saltier food after we take it. We use a little and get what we need. Protein types, as well as people who drink a lot of water above the norm of 0.033 liters per kilogram of body weight, need more salt. If you drink a lot of water, you wash your minerals out of your cells. And you fall into deficit. It is also important whether you drink coffee or other dehydrating drinks. For each coffee we should drink 500 ml of water above the norm for our weight. But we will discuss this in detail a little further.

People with low blood pressure, who often feel dizzy or have palpitations, can add a grain of coarse sea salt to their water. It doesn't have to be salty! Why? Salt affects the level of electrolytes in the body. When they are low, the things described above happen. This is a trick that is used by athletes in heavy summer training.

Bags Under the Eyes and Facial Swelling

Our achievements always match our ambitions.

Andrew Kurpatov

Why and how to get rid of them?

Let's start with "What does bags under the eyes mean?"

1. Poor lymphatic circulation! Imagine the lymph as the maid cleaning the rooms. She comes to take the empty glasses and plates, to make the bed, to put everything in order. She takes the night pot and throws it away, cleans the walls of the children's drawings, removes the empty bottles after the crazy party. However, if there is no key for some of the rooms and she stops coming in for a day, for two... for a week... for a month... the rooms become unusable. This also happens to our body. The lymph stops cleansing the cells because there is severe swelling, toxicity or something else that impedes its circulation. If we lead a sedentary lifestyle, then the rivers in our body (blood and lymph) are not fast but are like a swamp.

2. Weak muscles! Everyone knows that if they want a tight ass or a six-pack, they have to weight train. And how many times have you trained your face?

    Yes, exactly!

    We are born with copied cells of our mothers. If they have tight muscles, their children will have it too (but we will talk about this in detail in another article). If you were born tight, it doesn't mean you will stay that way! As well as if you are born relaxed – you can always tighten up! You have to work on yourself. Bags under the eyes are an indication of a weak eye contour. This is not just a cosmetic issue!!! The muscle around the eye is one of the three round muscles in our body (eyes, mouth, labia). It is connected to the muscles that hold the eyeball. If it is weak, they are weak too. Eye problems begin – astigmatism, diopters, curtains, etc. We will soon talk about the 58 muscles in the face and how each hang on the previous one. The eye contour depends on the condition of the forehead. If our frontal muscle is relaxed, it is not able to pull the next ones properly. So, one works at the expense of the others – but not for long.

Either it relaxes or overworks itself and the problems start again.

3. We ate white salt, sugar, white flour, gluten or dairy products! If you haven't logged in to my site. Get in! semma.bg. Up in the free category see the poster "Beautiful face." These are four people describing skin problems after consuming these products. You see the problem – you know what not to eat! In this case, the main problem with them is toxicity, fluid retention and processes they cause. In the morning we are swollen, the rings are stuck to our fingers, we need a ton of makeup to hide the damage.

How to get rid of it?

1. We go to bed early so that the body can regenerate. Sleep between 22:00 and 06:00 in the morning is vital. Four hours we regenerate physics, 4 hours psyche, we produce melanin and many other hormones. If we lose the hours between 22:00 and 24:00 we lose our health.

2. Reduce or stop the consumption of white salt, sugar, white flour, gluten and dairy products! Look at the pictures about the consequences of their consumption and find out what is bothering you.

3. Use the 3-minute facial wash technique and the 40-second cream application technique. If you don't know them, write to me, I'll share them again.
4. By doing a drainage massage. I personally use magic massage with spoons.
5. By training the facial muscles for 16 minutes 3 times a week for 3 months. Then you will not have a lymph problem. You will forget about dark circles, bags, pimples, wrinkles, loose contour, double chin and whatever else you can think of.

   Remember! The workout only works if there is no swelling in the face! I wish you a magical day, Wonderful!

Success is the opportunity to wake up and go to sleep being able to do in between whatever you really like.

Bob Dilan

I Want to Lose Weight! Cardio, Strength Workout, or Starving?

How to choose the right workout? Strength, cardio, hunger, diet, sweat, deprivation.... Oh, NO!!! I better stay fluffy. They will just call me "fluffy"!

In fact, we make it look scary. This is the result of thousands of diets and improper sports. Either we freeze in a certain phase, or we gain double the weight. Why?

Let's see – strength or cardio training? Like the typical woman – I love two in one.

Cardio – raises the pulse. We have a large energy expenditure in a short time. Usually 45 minutes (the workout itself). If we make it circular (interval in which things are repeated), then from 2 to 8 hours after training we may have increased energy and caloric expenditure. You will have a huge result in two months. You can lose 10–15 kg in a month. Then there will be a plateau. If it's pure cardio – you throw away water and lymph, liquid fat and you can burn muscle. Feeling is very important here. And let's keep in mind – The body gets used to it! It's not stupid! The workout must be changed.

Power – a month or two will be stagnant. You will even start to swell slightly. It is written everywhere in the textbooks – the muscles utilize the most energy. More muscle – more calories burned. Here the muscle is hungry for 12 to 38 hours. Accordingly, the metabolism is enhanced. In 10 years of work and 20 more sports, I saw the following: if a woman trains only strength training, she gets hard cellulite. Muscle begins to grow and fat enters it. Then to break such a structure is "mission impossible." In strength training, I don't like the fact that you inflate a lot. The muscle becomes bulky and if you stop, you become soft as jelly.

What role does oxygen play in the whole picture?
Scientists determine the energy expended in our body by the amount of oxygen the body consumes. More oxygen – more calories burned. Accordingly, the additional Post-Workout Oxygen Consumption (PWOC) determines how many calories we burn at rest.

Are we burning muscle or fat? Every second article is: "No starvation or efforts – 10 kg per month!" The problem is that the faster they go, the faster they return. Everyone associates becoming slim with weight loss! For me, the scales are the worst. I weight myself 3–4 times a year. Half a kilo of fat is about 4,500 calories. If we lose weight fast, it's usually water, muscle (we eat ourselves) and a little fat. Here I exclude people who have to lose 30–50 kg. It is normal to start quickly, because they have a lot of water retention and stagnation! If you need to lose 5 to 20 kg, the norm is 0.5 kg per week. WHY? Because by burning fat, you build muscle! When I don't work out, I am 47 kg. When I work out – 53–55 kg. As in the second case, I have 6 cm smaller circumferences in the thighs, pelvis and abdomen. One kilogram of fat in volume is as much as 4 kg of muscle. Here I give an example with Doni – in 29 days she did not drop any kilos, but she lost 16 cm in her legs, hips, abdomen!

And my favorite – hacks. Translated – cheating the system. If you've played games, you remember the codes. You write the code or go directly. You save time! Nature created women as multitasking beings. We do many things at once. As a typical woman, I am very lazy. When I was told that I should either stop training or do 6 types of training, 3 times a week, I said to myself "are they crazy?"

And I hacked the system!
How?
If we breathe properly, we are like a calorie burner. Something like "crazy with the machine gun," but in our favor. We burn a

lot for a short time. We increase the metabolism. By moving fast, we clean all the fluids (lymph, blood, liquid fat, etc.). The blood carries the smoothie to Every cell and we eat. If we breathe really well, it carries oxygen. It enhances regeneration in tissues and organs. It irrigates the brain. It releases hormones that are responsible for the constriction of blood vessels and their elasticity. Varicose veins and bad memory get healed. If we have opened the diaphragm well and we breathe, breathe, breathe, then we press the spine back and straighten the distortions, and vice versa, if we stand straight and breathe, then we train the diaphragm.

This is a muscle that 90% of the population does not use!

We need the diaphragm to take a deep breath. If we breathe like this in training, we learn to use it for the remaining 23 hours of the day. So, we burn more calories all day! We become stable, upright and self-confident like "show-offs."

Here we put the circuit strength training. If you always train at 80–100% – you feel the muscle split. You feel the burning and the maximum extension in the muscle – it will grow. Accordingly, you will burn up to 38 hours, not like pure cardio. Thus, people who train four times a week train every 24 hours and further increase the expense. They rest for two days and train in the evening, this makes about 56 hours. 56 minus 38 hours makes 18 hours a week (from 168 hours), in which they burn less than usual. Or 158 hours, in which we expend many times more calories than 18 hours. In this case, you do not need calorie deprivation. If you stand up and have no hunches, the increase in metabolism is many times more than 168 hours during the week! Because there is nothing to slow it down. You work the whole body, not a muscle group!

Thus, with one strength cardio workout with proper breathing and positions, you burn 1,800 to 3,000 calories per hour. The daily intake is about 1,500 calories. And if you are on a diet of about 1,000... Why should we deprive ourselves when we can burn them in 30 minutes? And even if you stop working out not a gram will come back!

The conclusion – you need both. You can do cardio and strength workouts separately. But you need both! One feeds you with air, the other with strength. And if you manage to combine them – you will be the best.

And if you want to see it in practice – follow me on Facebook! Write to me to save a spinning bike for you and come to a free workout. Find out what it is and then use it in your workouts!

And here someone will say, "Okay, but summer is coming I have to lose weight in two months." Don't lose weight from summer to summer! Keep yourself in good shape for yourself! And not to show off with the new swimsuit! The body has a memory! If you gain weight every winter because you eat a lot then, even if you don't eat a lot, it will take you two winters to wean your body from gaining weight. The clock in you is ticking! If you gain weight for two or three winters, you will gain the next one as well. Teach it that it does not need to gain, because you will always give it what it needs!

Have a lovely day, Wonderful!

My Sweet Phone Near My Bed

Nowadays we are all obsessed with our phones! Everybody is taking pictures of their children. When I click on Facebook or another social network, I can learn everything about a person. We upload our lives on the Internet and forget to live!

It's like looking at things through glass! Glass that we put there **ourselves**. No emotion, no feelings! I regularly see couples taking so many photos together – eating, drinking. WHY? I know you and I know that things are not going well! You yourself told me yesterday how bad your relationship is and how you will separate. By taking them, you try to convince yourself that you have what you lack! If you had it, you wouldn't waste time sharing it, you would enjoy it!

We hold on to these phones as if our lives depend on them. We take pictures of our dinner, we take pictures of our pajamas, we take pictures of our children, we take pictures, we write... And then we don't have time to cook healthy for tomorrow and take it to work. We don't have time to read a book with the children! We don't have time...

At one of my performances in a big mall, I heard "**I have no time**" over 1,000 times, and I saw people going around the shops 5 hours later! One girl stopped to hear about the award. And when she realized what it was – **she has to train**, she said "NO WAY! I have no time! And don't you have a page where I can read?" Yes, of course we have! Judging by the fact that she had about 30 kg to lose, but she was in stretchy pants and extensions, do you think she would sit down to read about her health? But the fact that she is on the phone is okay! And before I start talking trash about the whole world, let me say something on the subject.

The phone! What does it do?

Now you know what it does is steal our time. Time you can't buy. Time you can't bring back! Time you will lose in someone else's fictional life.

I exclude valuable pages here! BUT how often are you in such pages? Pages from which you do something after reading!

What else? The light! I have written four articles about blue light, how regeneration stops, how it ages you, how it wears you out, and 1,000 other consequences. And here you will read about it as well.

Something else? You look down at the phone. You lower your head. You have a feeling of inferiority, of depression, of insecurity. The bulb in your head is on! Danger! You start storing fat for the hard gloomy days! Hello big ass and cellulite. Tissues and organs age. Problems with lymph and swelling of the face, limbs and the whole body begin.

From the posture and the lowered head, you twist the spine! Your back is in the shape of a "C" and the total pressure increases many times more.

The eyes? What happens to them? Hello, astigmatism and diopters! Wrinkles on the face? Easy work. Look around! Anyone sitting on their phone has a tick. If you look at it for 2–3 minutes you will see how it makes the same movement, the same wrinkle activates several times a minute. And then?

And the cherry on the cake – the radiation! You've watched thousands of videos of a phone blaring in someone's pocket or frying eggs between two phones. And what did you do about it?

At the last International Water Conference, brain surgeon Jack Cruz told my brother that he would not talk with a phone next to his head for anything in the world! "I do brain surgeries all day, believe me!" He only speaks with headphones.

The phone should be as far away from your head as possible.

I used to carry my phone in the pocket of my jeans. For a year I had polycystic ovaries. Many customers have observed a relationship between where they carry the phone and tumor formations. Right pocket – cyst of the right testicle. And much more. The headache is regular!

What do we do? We go to bed and stay on the phone. Instead of calming the body without blue light, we wake it up! Blue light is like slap after slap. Produces cortisol. It wakes us up. Finally exhausted – we fall asleep. We put it next to us. It irradiates up to 6 meters. We irradiate ourselves; we irradiate our children!

And if you ask me, what does this have to do with beauty? If you have a tumor in your head, you will hardly be beautiful! You will hardly have hair from radiotherapy! You will hardly have good coordination! You will hardly be happy! You will hardly live long and fruitfully!

Forget about the regular "from tomorrow." Go and buy headphones. Put them on the phone and don't unplug them! You yourself don't know what's going on in your head, how can anyone else know! Put the phone on airplane mode or preferably in the evening turn it off. Leave it in the other room! Not by the bed! And now your brain says, "But it's waking me up!" Buy an alarm clock! It costs one lev. How much does your health cost?

It's up to you!

The Secret

Meaningless life is not worth living.

Socrates

I love it when we do self-massages or breathing. Then all the secrets come to light. Everything hidden in us wants to come out. And the secret itself is not the problem, but the way it grasps us in its claws and doesn't let us go. How we hide it inside ourselves without even knowing it! We put up our own bars, we enter a cage in which the padlock is inside and we have the key within. And yet we make ourselves the scapegoat.

Muscles are like books. They very carefully keep the emotions to themselves. And so, they keep us tied up. In order to protect itself and us, our body closes the emotion in a muscle. Tightening, plexitis or pain do not have to be caused by exercise. It can be from emotion.

This is seen in our daily lives. For example, as we breathe and saturate with oxygen, we will feel how in certain places, as if the blood does not want to pass! I was like that. When I was on holotropic breathing, I felt excruciating pain and cramps in my thighs. When I was little, I was very sickly. I was constantly getting injections in my legs 3 times a day. The nurse drew shapes and animals on them to distract me. I was so scared I couldn't relax my muscles. Just by remembering I was tightening them. Until at one point I couldn't let them go. Years passed; the memories faded. There is only one happy memory left, how my father and I came out of the entrance after another injection at the First Polyclinic in Burgas, he carried me in his arms and a man in a Zhiguli stopped him. The man had locked his keys inside and asked that I go through the trunk and unlock it. My legs hurt so much, I wanted them not to be mine, but of course, Ema went through the trunk and opened the car!

Over the years, I often got something like cramps in my thighs in the evening. I woke up shouting. I drank magnesium – and nothing. Until the holotropic breathing explained to me that I should relax. That this is a trauma, that this is an emotion. I began to think a lot about what I had experienced. I started doing self-massages, which hurt indescribably! You put a ball on the sore spot and press it downwards. The strange thing was that after the massages I felt depressed, I was crying, feeling sad and miserable. I was crying, and I didn't even know why. I wanted to eat all the chocolate and ice cream in the store. After 2–3 weeks of such emotions, my muscles relaxed. Now I can crush them and not even feel the pressure.

In the same way, I see in training who likes to control. Dominant people like to tighten their arms! All of their veins pop out, and even when you tell them to relax, they **cannot**! If you breath repetitively and you saturate with oxygen and then start feeling tension in your arms – yes, this is control! You can rub them to relax the muscles. **But first of all, you need to give freedom to others and yourself!** The world will not end without you. Usually, these people can't do without a phone. They want to know everything – when, how, why.

I had a client who was suffocating when we were doing the breathing. Strange right? You are saturated with oxygen and you are suffocating! This suffocation is fear. It can be like tightening. As strong pressure in the solar plexus. Like tightening a hoop around our neck. This is a fear we have once experienced. It may be in our childhood. It could just be someone's cry! We may be startled! Or it could be something that scared us to death! To overcome it, we need to focus on it and relax. If it is heavy and hard, imagine it soft and light, like a feather. If it tightens around your necks, imagine it as a warm hug. If it's cold, make it warm.

Another case is when I hear: "I feel pain in my ovaries!" The first time I said to myself: "How can your ovaries hurt you from breathing?" Then I talked to her. She told me she has no sexual desires, as if she has a stone on her stomach. Or that she feels something tightening. I started thinking about my first breathing. It was like my uterus was 99% pressed. I never felt pressure like this before. I was told it was a trauma again. During the long conversation and analysis, it became clear that it was due to birth stress. I gave birth to my two girls naturally. I went without dilation and they gave me oxytocin. In 30 minutes, I was about to die. I screamed, yelled, bit my hand to blood. For the next 6 hours it was pain I never felt before. And the moment I thought I was going to die and I couldn't do it anymore, they said to me "Push!" The women next to me looked in amazement. One came with 9 cm dilation and was there just to get examined! The other one was solving a crossword puzzle quietly and meekly without flinching. It was as if she was drinking her tea at a sunny window. This relieved me, and the next time there was no pressure problem.

I decided to tell the woman that it was similar with her. They used forceps to remove the baby. The fear of losing it is terrifying! The fear was so ingrained in her that her female chakra had closed. She had no desire for sex. She was overweight right in that area – belly and muffin top.

Rigid tendons mean limited movement. Cramped muscle means difficult and slow circulation of blood and lymph. Lack of nutrients: aging of tissues and organs. The body contracts because the muscle pulls it to one side. A shrunken body means the release of negative hormones. If there are any negative hormones in the body, we are in a mode of accumulation and storage. We gain weight. Slow atrophy. Wrinkles. Drooping skin. Cellulite... I don't even have to go on.

How you can help yourself?

Buy a ball. It can be a massage one, it can be for golf, for tennis... whatever. But it must be a BALL! You can start with a softer one and after a week or two – with a harder one. Find where it hurts. But do not press gently with one finger. Press with your thumb as if you want to pierce inside. You can place the ball and lie on top of it. It hurts, doesn't it!? Think about when it hurt and you didn't pay attention to it. Do not move. Stay on top of it. Stay in the most painful spot! You think you can't do it anymore? You can have at least another 20 seconds! Slowly remove it. Stay on the ground. Feel how you relax. Feel how relieved you are. How free you feel in your skin. Do you feel the emotion? It doesn't have to be right away. It may be in an hour. It could be in two. If you want to cry – cry. Cry as loud as you can. Get rid of what was holding you back. If you want to shout – SHOUT! Play your favorite song and shout your lungs out!

Every week I scream together with my children! We put something in the car, at home or in the hall. And on the choruses, we go: "3,2,1 AAAAAAAA-aaaaaaaaa" until we run out of breath. You don't have to hide everything in yourself. Nobody cares that you carry three suitcases with sad memories. The memories are past!

Choose to live in them or here and now!

Act, Fairy! Get rid of the suitcases! Be light as a feather! Be yourself! Not a copy of other people's mistakes!

Time is limited so this is why you shouldn't lose it by living somebody else's life. Don't allow the noise of others' opinions to silence your inner voice. And most importantly – get the courage to follow your heart and intuition.

Steve Jobs

How to Prevent Ourselves
from Getting Cancer

All living things on the planet have a negative electric charge. Every living grass and plant, even the small streams and springs, have a minus 450 charge. The human body is -70. Every day our body is attacked by thousands of free radicals – some we take with food (water, fruits, vegetables, meat, pills), others through the skin (water, synthetics from clothes, creams and ointments), others through the air we breathe (gas evaporation, etc.).

What exactly are free radicals? Have you heard in chemistry classes about cations (+) and anions (–)? The cations without a companion are the free radicals that chaotically collide in everything, looking for their opposite in order to calm down. It's like a woman whose husband hasn't come home at 3 in the morning.

Imagine someone pushing you all the time and not letting you concentrate on your work! 90% of our energy will be entirely focused on how to avoid, calm or block it.

Who do free radicals actually hinder? Our cells.

Imagine a bubble with two more in it. The big bubble is our cell with a membrane that protects it from the outside in and vice versa. One little bubble is the mitochondria – the energy plant. The second little bubble is our DNA. And in between all this, there are hundreds of pluses that chaotically push everything on their way like a soccer crowd looking for trouble.

They crash into walls, scratch and break, blow up important things in the factory and the energy produced there is not enough. Crowd-fighting sections are being made, and the energy needed to maintain the shields (immune system), the army (white blood cells), the one responsible for generators, fuel, air and all other systems, drops to 50%. The entire ship is in danger of sinking. Suddenly, one of the **free radicals** finds a gap and manages to enter the control panel (DNA). It changes the lights from red to blue and the veil – a cell with new DNA. The ship's sensors detect an intruder, encapsulate the cage and throw it out. And so, a cell that could live, for example, 2 years, dies in 2 days.

The body begins to self-destruct and there comes cancer. If the excretory and lymphatic systems do not function well, this spreads and segments begin.

How do we get enough anions (minuses) to neutralize free radicals?

It's very simple. Eat more raw food! Why? There is nothing accidental in nature. Fruits and vegetables ripen, fall to the ground and after 2 days have already rotted to feed the soil. They will either be eaten or will be fertilizer for new fruits. From its detachment to 48 hours after that, i.e., from -450 charge everything starts to lose its negative particles little by little and acquires positive ones (from alive it becomes dead). Only humans consume dead food. Everything else kills to eat it now. After each heat treatment, the food loses its negative charge. Each roasted nut is a carcinogenic ball. Each non-soaked nut is an inhibitor that stops the release of your hormones (growth, development, happiness).

The animals drink water from springs and streams with a charge in nature -450, we drink bottled or from the tap with a charge of +250. And instead of recharging, we become even more exhausted.

Most of the energy in our lives the body loses in the processing of water and food. That is why it is very important to eat a small amount of high quality food.

Here comes the original source of vegetarianism. The first vegetarians were raw foodists. All junk food contains these things. But when we read such stories, the reaction is usually,

"Wow, this is a miracle" or "He was lucky," "God loves him and has heard his prayers," and so on. Raw food means a lot of free anions (negative charge) that keeps us alive! We have all heard or read the legends of Atlantis and the living crystal that keeps them alive! The living crystal is the negative charge that holds us like "four-bar batteries."

Everyone chooses how and how long to live! Everyone chooses what to give their attention, their money, their time, their energy to! Eat a handful of value, not quantity! I have already written many articles on how to make our food with a lot of anions and reduce the intake of cations. Just read the book until the end.

Start copying what you like. Copy. Copy. Copy. And you will find yourself.

Yoji Yamamoto

A Goodnight Glass of Wine

Feel the warmth of the fireplace, watch the fire play. It's as if thousands of fireflies are racing. Look out the window – snow is falling outside. The ground is frozen, only the song of the wind can be heard. Go back to the room. Feel the soft warm carpet beneath your feet. Look at your hands. Smell the red wine. A bouquet of sensations slides down your palate. How do you feel? You relax in the chair, lift your feet up on the cozy velvet stool and it is as if the world is perfect!

And why not with a cup of aromatic tea? Everyone that I start a consultation or workout with tells me how much they like a glass of wine in the evening.

The biggest revenge is great success.

Frank Sinatra

Why?

Because it relaxes you. Because you feel the lightness in your muscles. It seemed to clear the picture. The brain stops cycling in our busy lives and problems. The muscles relax.

We talked to Didi yesterday and she told me: "I love a glass of red wine so much! For a week now I have been recording what, when I eat and observing myself. I came to the conclusion that when I drink half a glass, the next day I have bags and swelling under my eyes. I already enjoy a glass of wine only on the weekends."

Another example: Vancheto. She no longer drinks the glass of wine that accompanied the dinner and her face shows visible cheekbones.

Third example: my father. They had been testing him for months. And he said, "When I drink whiskey, everything gets better. I see well. I read without glasses. It's a pity they don't let you drink." He felt much better when he had alcohol in his blood.

And now I will share with you why! In our daily lives we tighten our muscles. From the hunching and the incorrect posture, we do not stress them equally, and some work at the expense of others. That's how we tighten. We use 40–50% of our muscles, the rest are like on eternal rest. By tightening them, we do not let them go. Tighten your fist. Now try to put your finger through it to your palm. You can't, can you? The fist is the muscles. And the fluids in your body are your finger. Lymph and blood do not circulate.

You don't cleanse! You don't feed! No oxygen! The muscles are in spasms

And you don't have to feel cramps to know they're cramping. Grab your leg and press your thigh on the outside. Press hard! Stick your finger in it. Another way is to lie on one side on the ground on a small tennis ball. Feel how there are places where you can barely touch and the whole leg shrinks. Now find the middle between the nipple and the shoulder, and press! It hurts, doesn't it? Now run two fingers in front of and behind your ears. Strong! Now over the ear. Find a point just above the ear. Now insert the knuckles of your fingers at the end of the jaw. Slightly in front and under the ear. Go to the eyebrows now. Strong! Press the knuckles. Let's go up. The base of the hair above the eyebrows. Press hard. This is how to treat every muscle in a "Get rid of stress" technique. Some give up cigarettes after that, others give up alcohol.

Drinking alcohol expands the blood system and relaxes the muscles. This is how food gets to it. But another issue comes. When you have alcohol in your body you are in a storage regime. This is how everything that you eat makes you fat. You cannot regenerate. You relax but it is not real. The processes you need to happen when you are relaxed are missing!

You can achieve the same with self-massage and proper breathing. Breathing should be 24 hours, not one workout! But in the beginning, choose moments to think about how you breathe! Open the diaphragm. On our site there is a FREE campaign: "Stand Yourself Up in 6 Weeks." Register and go for it. From the very beginning we give you a breathing exercise! The self-massage is with a ball, a small tennis ball or another. The goal is to relax a muscle, to clear it and feed it! Why do you have to drink a glass of wine to relieve yourself for an hour and fall asleep, when you can feel like that 24 hours/7 days a week/31 days a month/365 days a year?

Take care of yourself! Don't turn your body into a dump! Turn it into a machine! And I'm not just talking about muscles and relief! This body will be with you from beginning to end. It can do a lot! The question is where do you set boundaries for it! Your body is the perfect machine created by evolution.

Take advantage of it!

Use it according to its designation! Find what it can do!

You will surprise yourself with what your body can do!

It's your turn!

Freedom is not worth having if it does not include the freedom to make mistakes.

Mahatma Gandhi

A Great Day

I will admit that before the children were born, I had forgotten what the holidays meant! I used every non-working day for myself, or to catch up with work while no one was bothering me! My daily life dragged me like a funnel, from which I could not get out 24 hours a day/7 days a week. "Holiday" in my head is equal to a stolen day in which to catch up.

After I gave birth, I started studying again. What does Baba Marta, Christmas and all other **non-working** days mean! And I realized that no holiday is a random date! No custom is just like that. I don't know if it's weird or sad that the customs have survived, but people have forgotten why and what they mean. And now I will give you an example.

Easter is a holiday of eggs and salt.

All winter we only waste the accumulated stocks from the summer. We only eat dead food. We lose minerals and trace elements. Spring is coming and we are becoming very irritable. Every second person is sick and snorts. The weather is strange – in the morning it snows, at noon – rain, in the afternoon the sun shines. The body has difficulty adapting. And we are acidic not only emotionally, but also within ourselves. We eat sweets because our energy drops. We eat a lot of white flour and salt.

Why do we get sick? Because we are acids! Why are we acids? Because we eat dead food. Why do we eat dead food? Because it is winter and almost nothing is alive. "Alive" does not mean that your steak jumps on the plate and that the vegetables and fruits are torn off within 48 hours before you eat them.

Why do fasts come? What is the meaning of fasting?

Becoming alkaline!

The unexamined life is not worth living.

Socrates

Microbes and molecules harmful to us live in an acidic environment. Do you see the logic already? Fasting is not for you to deprive yourself of food! Fasting is about eating something that is not cooked! The problem is that nowadays when we fast, we do not eat live food, but cook it again. Anything that has undergone heat treatment is dead! Whether it's steamed, fried, roasted, boiled or whatever. If I boil you, I guess you won't be alive? Or steam you... it will hardly be any different! To turn acidity into alkalinity, you need live food.

That's why everyone gets sick in those seasons when there is no live food. Why is the doctor's office almost always free in the summer? Because we only eat live! Fruits and vegetables are in abundance!

There is almost no protein in live food! Excluding soaked nuts. In reality, we deprive ourselves of it for the period of fasting. If we are a carb type, it's great! But if we are protein, we fall into a deficit and after the end of fasting we gain weight. Why? The body panics at the lack. When we start eating protein again, it harvests it for rainy days. It does not know when we will want to starve again. That is why fasting is not for everyone.

Why do we eat eggs after fasting? And with salt! Eggs are protein! This makes up for the lack of protein. And why with salt? Coarse sea salt is composed of 72 trace elements. This is how you get the microelements that you were deficient in during the winter.

The problem today – we do not eat sea salt! What is the difference between salt, sea salt in a salt shaker, Himalayan salt and coarse gray sea salt? If you do not know, now I will tell you: if you want to be healthy, buy the last one. It is gray and greasy in the package; it is not sold in salt shakers. If you still don't understand why – go back to the beginning of the book.

If you do not feel well when fasting, eat cooked beans for protein and lots of fresh food. Soak nuts and eat them alive. Your goal is to cleanse. To become alkaline. And then recharge! You don't have to fast to achieve it. If you're like me, eat meat. But eat some meat and a lot of live food. Not cooked! I will share something here. Ever since I've been training and measuring with the metabolic age machine, I've been shocked by the results! Women 25 years of age have 58 years metabolically. The average life expectancy of a woman is 66 years of age. They are 25 and their body thinks that they have only 8 years left. It's sad! Slim, exercising women have critical liver obesity. From type 12, we enter a very dangerous zone at a value of 7. This means that while drinking your coffee you can have a stroke, out of nowhere. Think about yourself! Think about what you do and HOW you do it! Does it help or harm you! And if you decide today to compromise on something, don't compromise your life!

Instead of writing a book worth reading, better do something writing a book about.

Benjamin Franklin

Trick Your Brain! How to Hack the System in Our Favor

It is amazing how emotions impact the positions of the body. Have you noticed? And do you know that positions of the body impact our emotions?

Every emotion, every feeling is related to a body movement. They are accompanied by releasing certain hormones. And hormones boost this emotion – stress, happiness, sadness, depression, sleepiness... By releasing stress hormones, our motivation and confidence drops. Our body automatically droops the shoulders, chest is inwards, eyes are looking down. As if we are shorter than grass. And vice versa! If you are extremely happy, you feel your energy flowing and you can't even sit down. Lower your eyes, shrink your shoulders and you will see how you will instantly feel bad! You will become sad and will feel inner disappointment, guilt, a feeling of inferiority will come.

What if this is how you actually feel?

Everyone sets their own boundaries.

Richard Bach

Sit up. Raise your chin, eyes up high, straighten the back and the shoulders, jump up a few times. Feel your confidence! Feel how you have much more self-confidence than before! Feel your pulse! Feel your excitement! As if you are bubbling up!

You just produced the hormones of happiness yourself
If it's the end of the workday and you are tired but there is another hour before leaving and you feel like your energy is minus 200 of 10, then **Smile!!!**

Yes, you read correctly. Smile! The body does not recognize the true from the false smile. A smile means releasing endorphins! HAPPINESS! You will automatically receive a dose of energy! What does a 30-second smile cost you. Often, when my children are crooked, sleepy, or hungry, they begin to sulk. And if it's getting worse! I make them laugh. I stand opposite them and say something they will laugh at or say directly: "I challenge you! Smile at me and hold for 30 seconds." And it works. In half a minute they become like other children.

In my trainings and personal consultations, I aim to make people laugh every 15 minutes. As you know, if you laugh, you raise your energy. So, in the hardest part of the workout, it's like drinking a dose of energy. My trainings are all day for 6–8 hours. How will you survive if you only use your strength, but do not produce energy?! Have you been to boring seminars? After the second hour you fall asleep and a rumbling starts going on in the hall. Finally, it's good that you kept notes, because there's nothing left in your head.

Were you there at all?

That's why we commented on that topic when we talked about diets. We score an own goal! We want to be happy, but we stand hunched over and crooked. We feel bad for the candy we ate. What about that chocolate yesterday? Yesterday I saw a pimple on the bottom of Simonka's face. It had the typical pigmentation for sugar plus gluten. I told her, "You ate gluten." And she immediately said, "Yes, there were birthdays yesterday" and she began to excuse herself. Meaning: we believe that eating sweets is bad! We are filling up. We eat sweets quickly; we do not enjoy it. Then we have a sense of guilt. The body is shrunken and has stress hormones. We try to forget it. And if someone asks us, we immediately react with a defensive excuse. Not necessary! We ate – we ate. Why do we have to excuse ourselves? On the contrary, if you eat it anyway... **Enjoy it!**

How to help ourselves?

For starters – don't feel bad that you ate sweets! Think about what you ate before! That's the problem. It has not given you what you need. And the body wants to compensate with what you have taught it. Better eat something than nothing.

Stay upright. No matter how tired you are. If you shrink, work on the computer or on the desk hunched all day – you will not lose weight, no matter the diet. It's kind of like red light – a threat! You are hunched over – things are not okay! Store! Store! Store! Produce more stress hormones! Come on, come on, come on... no time! Winter is coming!

Produce more happiness hormone! Smile! Produce more motivation hormone! Celebrate every victory! HOW? Set easy goals! In two weeks – lose 1 cm from the waist. Clap, shout, rejoice.

And don't forget that whether the hen or the egg comes first doesn't matter! You have both a hen and an egg.

Whether you are tired and sad, you will hunch over... Or you will hunch over and it will make you sad, it doesn't matter. You will be sad! Will the smile come first and then the laughter, or will you laugh first, and then remain with a smile?

Which Hormones Prevent Us from Losing Weight and Which Ones Help Us?

Evolution knows what it is doing! We have memory encoded over the centuries in every cell. Whether we will use it is our decision. It's like a car. You buy it white, but you can always change its color, right? It will take time and money, but it will turn red! It can be shiny or rusty over time. It depends on how you care for it! So it is with the body.

The human body is like a ball of cables and wires. Everything sends signals and says "release this hormone," "I need the other one," "give me some oil," "turn on the lamp," etc. We have hormones that make us accumulate winter food for the hard days. We have hormones, which make us relax, we have hormones that make us cleanse, and they are all related to our mood, body posture and food.

The appetite panel is the hypothalamus. A corner of the brain that is responsible for the feeling of hunger. It's like a lot of drunk women in one place.

Some of them are:

Peptide YY – It is formed in the cells of the lining of the colon and controls the feeling of satiety. It is synthesized after each meal. If we ate value, this hormone reduced our feeling of hunger by 30%. It suppresses the secretion of the pancreas, bile and gastric juices and slows down the movement of food through the digestive tract. But if we read the fine print below the contract with the hormone we will see: if we do not go to the toilet regularly, how many times we eat a day minus one (2–3), then we do not have enough stomach acid to process food. We clog the intestines. We have a feeling of satiety and heaviness. The brain tells us to eat more because the stomach is empty. This peptide is stimulated by aerobic exercise as well as protein consumption.

Glucagon – A similar peptide. It is released immediately after a meal and stimulates the release of insulin. Insulin lowers blood sugar by regulating the metabolism of glucose and fructose in the body.

Leptin – More excessive weight, more leptin. If there is a lot, the appetite is low. It is artificially excreted by the consumption of proteins, vegetables and fats. BUT the body gets used to it and does not take it into account. That's why it's good not to wait until you weigh 60 kg to use this card.

Ghrelin – It is to blame for the yo-yo effect after stopping a diet. Its concentration in the blood increases before meals and decreases afterwards. If we have a disorder in its synthesis, we start gaining weight. When examining adults on a diet, the following dependence was seen: 17% weight reduction, 24% ghrelin increase. By stopping the diet, dieters will gain 24 times faster than before starting the diet.

Cortisol – The stress hormone. My favorite! If it is there, you're in storage mode! War is coming!

Thyroid hormones – If we do not have stress, then they are to blame for the weight gain. They are excreted in thyroid dysfunction. It is responsible for the feeling of heat/cold and, in particular, for always feeling cold. The feeling of heat exchange is disturbed. In these cases, you waste less energy on heating. Here it is important to monitor caloric intake. With this problem it is normal to gain 4–5 kg. But this is the beginning of an imbalance in calorie intake versus expenditure. The body lies and we start eating more. From there we gain more and it draws us. We release many of the hormones described above, the body changes, we bend over, a war begins inside us. Its outcome depends on us.

Female sex hormones – After the end of ovulation, the body adjusts to store fat. This way it will be ready for the future baby.

Women Are Unlucky – Evolution has taught us that summer has food; winter is in short supply. The man didn't matter. The woman is the one who has to survive the whole winter, bear the baby within herself, give birth and feed her child. Only then will the species be able to survive! That's why nature has decided men have one hormone to carry to the cage (to feed it) and one to clean (to export when needed). We women have 7 to carry and one to clean! So, in one month we become elephants who will not be able to use it in the next 7 months! Cool, ha?

What should we do?

Reduce stress and the cortisol levels – go to bed earlier, sleep 6–8 hours, breathe deeper, watch what you eat. Start moving more.

Produce more endorphins – stay in the sun, smile, be happy.

Produce more melatonin by sleeping from 21:00 to 01:00. And to control thyroid hormones – eat more seafood and consume coarse sea salt – unrefined!

Don't increase your carbohydrate intake, or rather stop it, when your period starts!

Aim at not just being a successful person, but a valuable one.
Albert Einstein

Raise your spirits:

Protein-rich foods (nuts) contain a large amount of tryptophan – an amino acid that is involved in the synthesis of serotonin (30 g of cashews, pistachios or almonds provide us with the daily dose).

In a 2013 study, the level of carotenoids of optimists was 13% higher than that of pessimists. Eat more orange vegetables (carrots, pumpkin, sweet potatoes, tangerines), which have strong antioxidants.

Foods with folic acid (vitamin B9) reduce depression. In one serving of red lentils there is 350 mg which is our daily intake.

The funny thing here is that a study published in *Neuropsychopharmacology* magazine shows that beer is also able to raise the amount of dopamine in the blood.

Don't stand in blue light! From sunset to sunrise, it is not good to stand in cold light (lamps, phones, tablets, computers, TVs). Programs and filters have already been invented for this purpose. If you do not use them, you stop the regeneration processes in your body!

I will share more on the topic later. Namely, how light affects us. Why we gain weight, why we grow old. How to fall asleep and get the necessary amount of sleep fast. The relationship between cancer and light! Emotions and everything else!

Poor Memory: How to Remember Like an Elephant and Have 100% Concentration

Poor memory equals poor blood circulation. And no, it's not a gene! Just because Mom or Grandma was like that doesn't mean you're like that. Remember the example: you buy a white car and you can always repaint it red!

Poor blood circulation comes from

1. Shallow breathing. And it comes from a weak diaphragm. If the diaphragm is strong, then we breathe deeply for 24 hours. Personally, for 26 years I have encountered only one diaphragm exercise! My brother showed it to you in the first video of our free campaign "Stand Yourself Up in 6 Weeks." Join our website www.semma.bg and watch it.
2. Hunching. When we are hunched over, in these places there is a pinching of the lymphatic and circulatory system. No nutrients, no waste cleaning. There is no way to be hunched over and able to breathe deeply. Accordingly, the blood is poor in oxygen! Without food and in a dirty workplace, who would want to work?

In the end, it all comes down to what we have in our blood! If we have oxygen and it reaches the brain, we will also have good memory and concentration.

And here I will tell you how to increase it even more.

Have you heard of baobabs? Yes, that big tree in Africa! Its fruit has a very pleasant lemon flavor. Thanks to the high content of vitamin C in a teaspoon of 52.5 mg it stimulates many processes in the body. It is no coincidence that when we get sick, we buy vitamin C from the pharmacy first! In addition, it contains calcium, potassium, fiber and vitamin B6. It has a very strong antioxidant effect. In other words, it neutralizes free radicals in the body and cleanses slag.

The ingredients of baobab enhance collagen synthesis. And, I hope, you know that it is a building block in our body. Thirty-three percent of the proteins in us are collagen fibers. That is why the skin tightens and cleanses. I even use it as a face mask. You can put it in water or homemade yogurt, or egg yolk, or tea... it depends on what you want to achieve. We stay like this for 20 minutes and wash if off. Collagen is also in the digestive system. Therefore, it has a good effect on digestion, increases metabolism, alkalizes (makes us a healthy alkaline environment in which bacteria and candida do not grow), strengthens our immune system.

But let's go back to memory. Due to its composition (fiber, iron, calcium, potassium, magnesium, manganese, sodium, phosphorus, zinc, vitamin A, vitamin B1, vitamin B2, vitamin B3, vitamin Bb, vitamin C) baobab affects the circulatory system! Helps with blood circulation. It cleanses the slag in it and it's as if you're seeing and breathing for the first time.

And now the second assistant – ginkgo biloba! It has been known since ancient times. It is no coincidence that all medications and supplements prescribed for poor memory and poor hydration are based on ginkgo biloba. It improves blood circulation and oxygen transfer in the body, thus helping to irrigate the limbs, brain and all organs. It has antioxidant action. Supports the good functioning of the nervous system. In other words, it calms us down. So, we don't think about 1,000,000 things by doing something. And we are present here and now. It is no coincidence that the tree is recognized as a symbol of longevity. It has existed for over 200 million years, and some trees live up to 1,000 years.

Baobab and ginkgo biloba complement each other. In the morning I usually get up at 5:30–6:00. I make tea with ginger, dandelion and other herbs. Then I drink warm water with baobab, ginkgo biloba and edible yeast and write an article. Edible yeast has a lot of vitamin B and calms the nervous system. My concentration is unshakable until 14:00. Then my individual training begins. As I move, my concentration rises again.

I personally used to take them from various acquaintances who I knew were taking their own supplements. For me, this means quality, because I know many people who do not consume their own products! And secondly, I don't like pills. I love tea, dried and crushed herbs. I take pills only if I know it is a pure herbal mixture, without being chemically or thermally treated. Today I import supplements myself, because they were not found in Bulgaria. If you enter semma.bg you will find what I use for myself, my family and my clients. So, I solved the issue with "we don't have it" when I order something.

Important: The fact that you will see a brand on the site does not mean that I support the entire brand! But only this product, which is available on the site!

I'm regularly told: "I don't know what you are taking, But I want yours!" Well, this is mine! Try it and after a while you will tell me how you feel!

Have a wonderful day, Lovely one!

You will never swim the ocean if you are scared of losing sight of the shore.

Christopher Columbus

For and Against Sugar

Yesterday the kids and I passed by a pastry shop – large windows, sun, pretty tables. They asked me to let them eat something sweet. I'm not a Cerberus! In my opinion, everyone chooses how to live and they are well aware of that. One is 2 years old, the other is 4 years old and they can make adequate decisions about their food on their own. We sat inside. In 40 minutes, many people entered. Pupils, students, families, retirees and everyone had something in common! Their appearance!!! They all had some form of acne. From fine to strong, combined with pigmentation! Their shoulders were weak, depressed and sad. Their shoulders were hunched over... Their mental state was "I exist," not "I live." The skeletal structure was distorted at 3 spots at least – knees, waist, shoulders. There was an asymmetry in their face. Something that annoys you and you want to adjust. Like a vignette sticker placed in the center of the windshield, not in the corner!

And I did not stay behind. I ate a cheesecake yesterday. Perfect combination of milk, white flour, sugar (the three white deaths in one!). In 20 minutes, my head would burst with pain! I had pains in my heart all day. Today I woke up swollen! 40 minutes later the children had small, fine pimples. And not because the cakes were old! No. They tasted wonderful and were very fresh. As a cake should be!

What does sugar do?

When we eat, food breaks down into components. One of them is glucose, which our body uses as fuel (bread, pasta, vegetables, fruits and grains). Glucose is used by our brain, cells, tissues and organs. Lactose follows. It is first encountered by every mammal. The third is sucrose. It is made up of 50% glucose and 50% fructose. Fructose was very rare before. It was in fruits, vegetables, honey. Now we find it everywhere. It is fructose that makes eating sweet. So, you can always find out if there is fructose in your diet. Today, more and more people are suffering from something serious. Scientists believe that fructose is the problem.

For example – 400 ml of apple juice contains about 9 teaspoons of sugar. In cereals per serving there are 7.5 tsp. of sugar. If you add a portion of yogurt – 18 g – 4 tsp. And here are 20.5 tsp. of sugar for breakfast. The body does not need as much sugar, especially refined. Evolution itself does not want it. The body stops producing energy by itself, waiting for the next dose.

When I don't eat sugar (dried fruits, juices, pastries, cookies, etc.), I am much more energetic. If I eat sweets, my body waits for the next dose, instead of just producing energy. And so, from dose to dose, if you don't take the dose, you get irritated and nervous. It's like a doll which someone needs to constantly wind to make it move. And how nice would it be if you didn't have a winding mechanism? You will be the one to decide...

Indescribable and priceless!

What happens when sugar gets in our mouths?

It is divided into two parts – fructose and glucose. Both enter the liver. Upon entering there, the glucose is immediately converted into energy or stored, something like a battery for later. In nature, fructose is rare. The liver cannot digest it. If glucose has already charged all our batteries, fructose is automatically converted to fat. And much of it remains in the liver in the form of white sticky gum composed of fat. And from there the risk of diabetes increases. The rest of the fat leaves, we gain weight and we are at risk of heart disease, heart attack, stroke, etc.

How does glucose affect the brain?

If it is stable, then our psyche is fine. If its levels are unstable and we consume it all day, its values vary. This is how we become mentally unstable. Emotions in us vary from extreme to extreme, the levels of stress hormones rise. There is a risk of depression, schizophrenia and many others. A manic feeling arises, which we confuse with happiness. But this is not happiness! It comes and goes, like tides. If our brain is happy at 5 units, eating sugar, we raise these 5 to 20. We release insulin to lower them. But we lower them to -15. Adrenaline is released, which tells the brain: "Eat something sweet" (because that's how we trained it). We eat and everything repeats itself. One moment we are happy. The next we are in a panic attack, we have worries, mental disorders, fears etc. (caused by the level of adrenaline).

If what I've said so far is interesting, watch it on YouTube – Сахар Фильм 2016 (That Sugar Film). It is an hour and a half long and everything is shown visually with an experiment and many explanations.

Read the ingredients. Everything that ends in -ose is sugar. Every day, the average person consumes 40 teaspoons of sugar without necessarily eating sugar. Each teaspoon is about 4 grams. There is no such thing as a good sweetener. Teach your body to produce energy for you itself! There was no sugar 100 years ago and we have survived. And you will survive!

Smile today so that everyone around you wonders what happened. If you convince them that you are happy, then you really are. The brain does not recognize the fake smile, produce endorphins without the need for sugar.

In a Child's Head

Today I talked to Geri and Tsveti about the behavior of their children. You will never see mine shouting, arguing, fighting! I'm not talking about manners! If a child does not want to go to bed at night, has difficulty falling asleep, cannot concentrate, shouts, runs, etc., it eats a lot of carbohydrates. Carbohydrates for children are like coffee for adults. Think about how you would feel if you were on 5 coffees? I'm not talking about white sugar and flour here. Judging by the fact that you are reading my articles, you should have already removed them from the diet! All foods that make the child aggressive, too energetic or wild are not okay for him. The change in emotions means spikes and drops in blood sugar! This means a constant peak and drop in insulin. Constant fluctuations give way to diabetes. This is one of the reasons we are so predisposed to it. From children until our last breath, we are constantly playing with our insulin levels! And this is not a joke!

Think about how many diabetics there are around you! You don't want your child to be one of them, do you? Every mother wants the best for her children! To be healthy, to be happy, to be loved! Remember when your child had a fever, how your heart broke and you couldn't catch a wink of sleep all night! What if this continues for a day or two? Don't play with their blood sugar!

Many mothers give their children dairy products for calcium. Dairy products are pasteurized. I really like the example of a piece of research in England. Three generations of cats. Two control groups. One eats only cat food. The other – cat food with pasteurized milk. In the third generation, no cat knows its sex! Everyone has rickets! They all have many internal problems, adhesions, tears and anomalies. DNA has mutated.

The generation cannot continue! This happens to our world too! Look around!

The problem with dairy products is pasteurization! It changes the DNA of the milk molecule. And the least of our problems is that instead of getting calcium, we lose it. The side effects are huge! Not to mention that animal milk contains three times more casein than human milk. It is responsible for the structure of your bones. The larger an animal, the more diverse and saturated its molecules are. Therefore, milk causes bone and joint changes. BUT we will talk more about this in other pages.

While we are small, we compensate but then the big issue comes!

So don't do it. It is surprising how easy it is for us to be healthy!

For example, if the child wants yellow cheese, it lacks fat and protein. If it wants cheese, olives, something salty and delicious – it needs minerals. And there are 72 trace minerals in coarse gray greasy salt. It doesn't come in a saltshaker and is not white!

If after eating the child is sleepy – it ate too many fats!

Some people complain about roses' thorns all their life. I am thankful they have them.

Alfonse Car

The same way food affects us – it affects the child as well!

Food equates to hormone release which equates to emotions.

Food determines the way we are!

Let me stay with somebody for 10 minutes and I will tell you what they eat without even knowing them!

I fell in love with people when I realized that they were not bad, but that they simply did not eat what they needed. At trainings they always laugh at me, how I have at least 2–3 types of food in my bag. Walnuts (fat), almonds or banana (carbohydrate), pumpkin seeds or steak (protein). My children are of a different metabolic type to me and depending on their mood I know what they need. So, I do not give them everything, but only what is necessary. And they are never crooked and nervous. In my opinion I don't have a client I can't tell to "increase this, decrease this." Only by skin and posture can you see what is not good for you and what is.

Take care of yourself! Take care of your children! And before you get angry at how your child behaves, think about what you gave your child to eat!

Have a day full of smiles, Lovely one!

Feel the wind in your sails. Move... If there is no wind, work the paddles.

Latin proverb

Breast Cancer

I've been thinking about writing about this for a long time, but I still didn't. And lately, I've been flooded with information about a campaign with this focus. The only thing I don't understand is, "Why is everyone fighting the outcome, not the causes?" Everyone is campaigning for a fundraiser, and no one is talking about why it's happening!

Well, today I'm thinking of giving you a different point of view. Today I will give you specific reasons for the appearance of breast cancer. They will not be the ones you find everywhere.

Let's start!

Cancer lives where there is no oxygen. It is a mutation in our cells caused by our daily lives, habits, food and the products we use. Nowadays, everyone has shrugged shoulders and is hunched over. Only a few stand straight as a pole. At least two people a day ask me, "How is your posture so natural?" In the workouts I do for 6–9 hours, I don't stand on one leg, I don't shrug or hunch over. That's what you have to do too!

When we bend our shoulders forward (as we are non-stop), we tighten the chest muscles. Remember the example with the fist and the finger?

Your fist is the muscle in your chest. Your finger is lymph and blood. The first cleans the garbage, the second brings food and oxygen. If you are tight non-stop, there is no way to clean and feed. The muscle has no rest. There is no time for regeneration. There is no oxygen. Nobody wants to die. This is the meaning of evolution. You are adapting! No oxygen! **The cell mutates into one that lives without oxygen!** Cancer cell! As of 2017, there is already research on this topic and confirmed facts in England.

How many times have you squeezed your chest muscles? And no! I'm not saying the way your partner enjoys your breasts! The massage is done with a small tennis ball or similar. It is placed on the chest, aiming to reach the muscle, not the fat layer. It is easy for women with small breasts, it is more difficult for those with larger ones. Stand on a door frame or on the edge of a wall, position the ball and press. You do not pass through the alveoli and nipple. You only massage a muscle. It hurts a lot! You will hardly relax if you do it only one time. Massage the breast down, upwards, sideways, and up to the shoulder. Along the shoulder – nipple diagonal – you will find a spot that hurts a lot. This is the muscle that pulls your shoulders forward. The massage can be from 2–3 to 30 minutes. In the end stop and feel! Feel as if you dropped some huge weight!

Now think about how you stand. Nothing hunches you anymore. Stay upright. Otherwise, it will tighten again.

The second reason is shallow breathing. Think how you breathe! Whether it will fail to reach the blood or reach it but without any oxygen... it doesn't matter. Breathe deeply! Breathe with the diaphragm to the side. Stand in front of the mirror. Try to inhale and make your ribs go to the side. This is proper breathing. Like the gills of a fish.

Check your cosmetics! Have you read my articles on harmful substances? If you haven't read them, go to page 171! These substances cause cancer, cysts, kidney stones, hormonal imbalances, problems conceiving and various genetic changes. Check to see if they are in your shower gel, with which you wash every day, in the toothpaste, in the hand-washing gel, check all sorts of brands. Even if they are organic, I still haven't found one that doesn't contain them. Could this be why every third woman has cervical cancer, fibroids or cysts? Sodium lauryl sulfate (SLS) was invented during the war. It was invented to wash oil and rust from tanks. I don't think we're that dirty! And today they put it in every product! This is horror!

I know I gave you food for thought. And I believe that is enough for today!

The body should relax. And this does not happen with a glass of wine in the evening for health. This is done with a massage! And not with a masseur rehabilitator! A self-massage! Alone with yourself!

That's why I do a self-massage once a month for 3 hours with 12 people. Every muscle in the body is treated! From your ears to your toes! My goal is not advertising. My goal is for me to do this regularly. When I have a group my brain can't find an excuse not to do it. You can actually do it once a year. You can do it every week. It depends on how much you work! I train 5 days a week. And once a month is perfect for me. You decide!

You don't have to pay. Get together with friends. Arrange a place, date and time. No excuses!

Have a wonderful day, Precious!

Worry is unnecessary. If you can solve the problem you don't need to worry. If the problem cannot be solved, there is no point in worrying.

Mathew Rickar

Loose Joints and Flat Feet

Yesterday I had a consultation with yet another client who gave up doctors. She told me that she had "loose joints" by inheritance. So did her mother, so did she, and so did her eldest 4-year-old son.

What are loose joints? Joints that have more clearance in one direction. Why? One muscle is overstretched by constant contraction. The other at some point refuses to pull and relaxes. Thus, there is a strong pull on one side and a strong stretch on the other. One muscle shortens. With it, the tendons on this side harden because they do not shrink and stretch. And they are in constant contraction. They become hard. Like that gum under the desk standing there for a long time. On the other hand, the muscle is stretched and elongated. Tendons too. They are difficult to contract.

Imagine two cubes. If they are on top of each other, the base will be strong. If they are on one side and touch only their edge, little by little the edge will be rounded and erased. The construction is not strong. It's the same with the joints. Think of a time when you slept wrong. Or you overstretched something. How it hurts when you want to get it in the other direction. You want to bend your arm, but there is a strong sensation of needles, it hurts so much that it's impossible for you to do it immediately. Everything that stretches us too much does just that.

I loved yoga very much. When I was a student in Sofia, I had the opportunity to go to one of the best groups. She now organizes the largest yoga camps. It was pure coincidence. I was sent from university as compulsory physical education. But whenever they made us stretch our backs, I had pain in my vertebrae. It was as if they were clinging to each other and after that I had a burning sensation in that area. Immediately after the exercises I felt very good. I felt stretched, it would not be difficult for me to stand up. But after a few hours it became difficult for me to stand upright and vice versa – I hunched even more, and the burning in the vertebrae became awful. Many clients are overstretched by yoga. And not just from it. Gymnasts and ballerinas are the same. The body is displaced by strong stretches and the joints are bent more than necessary for proper posture. Thus, most often the knees move forward, as well as the waist, shoulders, head.

And back to the case. The loose joints were in the waist, shoulders, and the displaced head forward. It's not genetic! And it is not passed from mother to child. Nor from my client's mother. The transfer takes place in the "copy/paste" structure of the mother's cell to the child. But this is not a fundamental factor. Let's see. I told her:

"When you were little, you watched a lot of TV, right?"

"Yes."

"How did you sit on the couch? You sink into it, your back forms a C-shape, your shoulders and waist are clenched. The head protrudes."

"Yes."

"At school and university – the head is lowered. We write with shrugged shoulders forward. Looking at the phone, we lower our eyes. We stick our heads forward. We shrug forward. As we read a book, we put it on our lap, tilt our head forward. As we drive the car, we repeat the pose from the sofa and the TV."

"How is the posture of your son? Does he watch a lot of TV and is on the phone?"

"Ooooh, all the time!"

It's not our genes that distort us. But our everyday life. I pushed her where the muscles should have been tense and said:

"It must hurt here because they are in spasm."

And guess what? It hurt! The doctors had told her it was incurable! When my legs were almost paralyzed, the doctors told me it was because of lot of sports. They told me to stop dancing, to stop breakdancing, to stop running, everything! Sport is harmful!

When I took Iva to the doctor to see her legs, because she had a fallen arch, the doctor said, "It's normal." Use a flat feet insole. I used to have flat feet. And I cured myself with workouts! By myself! Then I didn't even know how I did it. I was just working out. I know the pains I had every evening from the insoles my parents made me wear. I was not going to do it to her!

What are flat feet? The muscles that are supposed to pull the arch are stretched and atrophied. They are not working! Putting on an insole is like putting plaster on a healthy muscle. What will happen? When we remove the cast, the imbalance will be on the other half of the leg. It will be weak; it will have no strength. We will need rehabilitation and movement to make it work. The choice is – to use insoles and atrophy completely or to work on it and be complete?

For doctors, what is not treated with a pill is incurable! There is no such thing as loose joints. Every displacement in the body is a consequence of a routine that we do wrong every day! We have developed a habit and do not even think about how we do it. We blame the genes, and they should only take 10% of the blame.

What do the pills do – relax the overstretched muscles. Like magnesium, for example. What does the massage do – relax the overstretched muscles! And who will tighten the atrophied muscles? Only you!

Life is wonderful! Muscles allow us such movements that other creatures on the planet can only dream of! I can't imagine life without movement! And I can't understand how anyone voluntarily gives up on that. Some do not live; they only exist for another 20 years! And they have their whole life before them! **Don't be this someone!**

How to Remove Deep Forehead Wrinkles

Beer – to drink or use… drink or use… This is the question!

During the last two weeks of individual training, I have been constantly asked, "How do you do it? One day you have such a wrinkle between your eyebrows, and the next you don't have it!" It's a fact! Ever since I knew how to get rid of them, I don't mind them! I remember my mom telling me: "Stop making faces, you will be ugly!"

I don't want to think about whether I'm showing emotion. I prefer to laugh, get angry and finally know how to get rid of them in a day. And what about you?

There is no magic pill! There is useful knowledge!

First: Relax! Massage your entire head. Stop for 30 seconds to a minute at each spot. You don't need a map of spots. I have a lot of videos where I talk about dark circles and bags. I'll show you how to rub your neck and shoulders. Do it! Make a fist and with the second phalanx (the second knuckle, the second joint) press everywhere gradually. Start at the chin and go over every millimeter of your face. You will be surprised how many spots will hurt you! **Hold on**! Don't skip. Pass around the nose, under the eyes, around the ears, around the eyes, forehead, up in the hair. After that, go to the scalp. Then at the back of the neck. Stop. What do you feel?

Your answer should be, "lightness." It's as if all the tension is gone. It's as tension left you alone for the first time. Feel the calmness. Feel the warmth. The lightness. It's nice, isn't it? Look at your expression in the mirror. It's as if you had the best orgasm. The corners of your mouth are slightly smiling. It's like you did something wrong.

Now intertwine the fingers of one hand and the other and place them on your forehead. Hold it stable so that the skin does not move. You can see it in the dark circles video as well. This is a forehead exercise. Look up. And now pull from the eyebrows as high as possible. Wait 2 minutes! Feel the burn from your eyebrow upwards. **You should not be able to wrinkle the skin! Hold still!** Otherwise, you will make more wrinkles!

Then put two fingers of one hand at the beginning of both eyebrows. And with the index finger of the other make a triangle between the eyebrows and slightly upwards with rotating movements. Feel the place getting warm and relaxed. Wait another 2 minutes.

For now, we did the basics. Now we need to iron the tablecloth.

We wash our face and put sour fruit on it. I love strawberries, kiwis, grapes. Maybe a tomato, a lemon, an orange. I take a strawberry and rub it in. I stay like this for 20 minutes, here is ANA acid, which exfoliates and regenerates. If you then see that you have flakes on your skin, just wash with a little baking soda and water and everything will be okay. You will see the pores shrink. The pigmentation is bleached. Fat is gone. Do this trick every day for a period of 14–20 days to renew the skin. And as maintenance – once a week, once a month. It's up to you.

Now the mask! Mix: 1 egg yolk, about half a banana, nutritional yeast (may be beer yeast), 1 tsp. baobab powder (available in organic stores or online), Q10 can also be added. Why?

The yolk is a protein. The base and the tissue are made of it. Banana hydrates and helps the structure. Yeast has B9. This is folic acid. It helps the plant in the cell to produce elastin, collagen and everything needed to prevent apoptosis (sagging). Or as I like to say – a landslide! During pregnancy we need a lot of folic acid. With it we help cell division. It's not just the baby's cells that divide! Vitamin A – is responsible for regeneration and is a powerful antioxidant. If we have vitamin E, we supplement. Q 10 is regeneration. Baobab – I love it! Lots of vitamin C, vitamin A, magnesium, zinc, potassium, calcium... advanced cocktail!

Many people tell me, "I drink collagen, I drink supplements, etc." The skin is the last destination they will go to! It is the red light that tells you something is wrong. But it will be fine when you fix the thing inside, so when you eat something and you know it's good for you, give it to the skin as well!

Now have a marvelous day, my dear!!!!

Be unique!

Not everything is invented already: the world is too wonderful for you to give up and sit back.

Richard Branson

Diet or Nutritional Plan

For the last two months I have not had a personal consultation that does not address the issue of food. So, I decided to shed some light on the DIET issue.

I don't know about you, but when someone tells me "don't eat bananas," I only think of bananas!

In the head of everybody DIET equals restriction, deprivation, sadness, depression, even grief. This is so encoded in our brains that it panics at the word itself. Why did I mention bananas? All my life until 5 years ago I tried not to eat bananas. The equation of banana = cellulite was stuck in my head. I don't want to have cellulite, so I won't eat bananas! And what was happening? I eat a banana every time, and then I feel guilty! Guilt means releasing stress hormones. If we have a high level of "negative hormones," those that do not help us feel good, then we store. The body adjusts to war and deprivation. Automatically, we begin to store each bite in a fat cell. We take it home for the upcoming difficult days! To achieve this goal, we do not need the 90-day diet! Just the thought going through our heads is enough! If I eat a banana and think about how I will have cellulite tomorrow, then I will have cellulite! Our thoughts determine which hormones to release.

And vice versa! You feel depressed, sad, you feel like cuddling with somebody, you suffer from lack of attention... **do you get me**? This is due to what we have eaten or what we think about. Your energy is dropping. And here is the key! You start to eat sweets and fast carbs. Your body wants to store. When stored, fat cells secrete the hormone of happiness – endorphin! And there you go – two birds with one stone! You will be happy, your ass will grow, fat cells will store for the difficult days you think of! **Everyone wins!** As they say in one of my favorite books that I read in ninth grade – *Winter Is Coming!* The brain has found a way to survive the winter, it is happy with what it has done, and you feel even happier! For short!

You are disappointed! Another diet does not work! And it all starts again! You can't lose weight because you are in a constant cycle. Disappointed with yourself!

Diet – a list of foods to eat! I really like to say "Eat this, if you don't die, you will lose weight!" This has stuck in my head opposite the word diet. Now all sorts of tests are very popular. They bring you foods that make you full. My most recent memory is what Doni shared a week ago: "I was told that I get fat from peaches. I eat peaches twice a year!" That is what I mean.

Why a nutritional plan based on metabolic type? – because it makes a habit. A good nutritional plan does not say "do not eat this." A good nutritional plan is not for a week, two or a month. **It is a way of life.** A life where you feel happy 24 hours a day. A life where you are 24 hours full of energy. A life where you do not feel restricted, you have no limits and deprivations. **A life where you eat everything and lose weight. A life where you feel satisfied with yourself.** A life where they come and ask you: "What do you use? I want yours!" I used to get angry when someone said to me, "Come on, eat just one piece, stop with your restrictions." I don't even want to eat what you offer me. I've already mentioned why we want sweets!

If you have a balance in your hormones, then you do not need sweets, and therefore no desire for some. It's like saying to a drug addict: "Come on, take a dose, what's the big deal." Because sugar, dough, milk is exactly an addiction. Your addiction!

To make everything clear to you, let's discuss **what a metabolic type is** and why it works this way.

All diets are based on fiber, water, protein. There are three metabolic types: carbohydrate, protein and mixed. Diets vary in composition depending on the metabolic type of the person who made them. They range from very light protein to very heavy. From very saturated carbohydrate to very heavy. Every person is different. If you eat according to a certain diet and you're still hungry, it's because you need heavier protein. If you do not have energy and you are still tired, or your protein is heavy, then you need a lighter one, or you lack fat. And it can be a combination of both. All diets are basically aimed at reducing calorie intake. The problem is that, again, everyone is different. And if you go from heavy and greasy food to light salads, you will lose weight because of deprivation and hunger. And then you will gain 2 times more.

I'm not saying diets are bad. In order to be shared on the Internet and to have millions of positive and negative reviews, it works one way or another. It works for those who are of a similar metabolic type to its creator. And it does not work for those who are of another metabolic type.

Stop seeking out the storms and enjoy more fully the sunlight.
Gordon Hinckley

If you only reduce the caloric intake in your diet, you increase the water of 0.033 liters per kilogram of body weight, you move more than usual – you will lose weight. The point is for the change to be positive in its entirety.

If you feel good in your skin, your diet works. If you are still dissatisfied and see only your shortcomings and not your achievements, then change your way of eating.

I have been happy with myself for the past 4 years. In these 4 years I was breastfeeding twice and I got pregnant once. Before that I was an instructor living in deprivation to be thin and slender. Now I eat everything I feel like eating. I eat bananas without having cellulite the next morning. How? I combined my previous knowledge with my latest training in London. I supplemented with what I learned from the Julia Sayfullina Beauty Academy in Moscow. So, I follow not only my metabolic type, but what my body tells me. I see when there is a deficiency of vitamins, iron, zinc, magnesium and many other trace elements that are visible on our skin. I don't want you to come to me for a personal consultation. I told you where I studied. There are thousands of materials. Read and act! Life is not endless and you decide for yourself the way you will live it. Will you just pass or will you experience it to the fullest!

And here is a secret: if you choose to live it to the fullest, don't do it in deprivation!

The first recipe for happiness is: avoid too lengthy meditation on the past.

Andre Maurois

Six Pack Abs: Yes, Yes, Yes ... No

I will ask you only one question – Do you want a six pack? It's beautiful, is not it? Admit it! It is not a question of whether it is difficult, but whether if somebody could give it to you just like that, would you like to have it?

Whoever says NO to me – I don't believe. But we have to be careful what we wish for!

Leave the looks aside. Let's look at the work of the abdominal muscles.

A tight stomach helps digest food. You probably know that the stomach has no teeth. How do you digest food? Tightening and relaxing. It can't tighten enough to squeeze it. The abdominal muscles help it. When we laugh, when we walk, in every accurate movement we use a different muscle chain in our body. It starts at one end (for example, our heel) and ends at the other end (fingers). Did you know that the place where your hair splits on top of your had can cause flat feet? We will talk about it soon! These are the chains. The abdomen is used for 24 hours. We must use it in every move. And the diaphragm works while we sleep as well – we breathe. There is really no second in which the abdomen is at rest.

Once it helped digest the food, it then pushes the contents towards the intestines. You must have heard about lazy guts. The problem is not in the intestines, but in the stretched lower abdominal wall. Once you have a big stomach – if you eat a lot, it stretches. Then there are the intestines – if you can't push the food, it ferments and poisons you. You're getting poisoned. It's like eating a freshly roasted steak or lentils with a steak kept out of the fridge for 3 days. The intestines swell and stretch. You hold feces. From there, the abdominal wall stretches.

How do we know if we are holding back? You have two bones on the side of your triangle. For some they are hidden, for others they are palpable, for some, they are visible. The distance between these two bones after you poop should be like a flat board. If not – there is more. How to remove it? By eating fiber and working on the lower abdominal wall. And no! This is not about lifting your legs.

What happens when we make a six pack from the navel to the ribs. We tighten the diaphragm. We stop breathing! The diaphragm must be loose. The abdomen in this area should be stretched, not tightened. And the diaphragm itself shall be trained separately. How? With breathing. With painful breathing! It hurts on the inside of the ribs, between the bones themselves. You want to stop breathing, but you can't.

The lower abdominal wall is responsible for our posture. It is responsible for the entire body – how we stand. Whether we have a problem with the back, knees, shoulders, head. Whether our waist is forward or backward. Look at yourself in the mirror. If you have a belly. If you drink a glass of water and you look like a "pregnant cockroach" in its sixth month. If your waist has a curve forward as if you are showing off your ass. If you tilt when you walk.

Then the lower abdominal wall is missing!

After giving birth it is zero! So far, there are 2 local exercises that tighten it. And you will see them only in corrective gymnastics. You can see them on our site if you sign up for the free "Stand Yourself Up in 6 Weeks" campaign. This is video tutorial number 2.

To work the lower abdominal wall, you must use either the chain in the body or you need to act locally. And these are not the pushups in the gym and on the Internet. They train the upper abdominal wall. You need sick pack abs from the groin to the navel, not from the navel to the ribs.

Love yourself! Love your body! Ninety-nine percent of women do not like their butt or belly. And they are interconnected. Fix one and you will fix the other.

Spend the day in love, Princess. May butterflies flutter in your belly and may the smile be glued to your face.

If you do the dishes, just do the dishes. Don't worry about anything else… We forget to enjoy the regular things from the day. We forget to see the beauty hidden in everyday life.

Julia Roberts

Together for 12 Years

Every day I see stories of people sharing about their long-term relationships – a year, two, three. They give advice on how to be in the relationship, what he or she wants and similar. And I started thinking. In September 2018 it will be 12 years since I have officially been with my husband. And April 2018 will be the non-official anniversary. I am a little confused, does the first time you had sex count or living under one roof?!?

I have two children and 12 years of married life. Is it luck? Faith? I don't think so. A lot of work on myself, thousands of mistakes and failures and as many successes.

I constantly hear about somebody seeking the perfect partner. And we don't realize that they will not come if we spend all day on the computer. In the first course I used to hear people wanting to meet Mr. Perfect! And we were joking that if they order pizza they might meet him. If you don't go, only he can come to you. But how great are the odds? And how great are the odds that he is a pizza delivery guy with 8-pack abs, tight ass, charming smile and a kind soul...

In 2018 everybody walks around looking at their phones! Children are playing on the playground 7–8 years old, and every child has a phone! I don't know, maybe I'm the mistaken one! But it doesn't look normal to me! Mothers take photos of their child's every move, dads play poker, billiard or the like while the child is screaming: "Dad, look at me!" As if we are not alive! And then somebody else is to blame!

And what did I learn after all? That there is no such thing as Mr. Perfect!!!

We create him ourselves!

We change ourselves to fit in with him! And then he is still not perfect! Because we are not perfect! Food forms our hormones;

our hormones determine what we are. Are we crooked, happy, sad, angry! Every time we compromise with our food, we compromise with ourselves! And we take it out on our close ones!

Before I used to be jealous, I was obsessed. "Where are you?", "Who is this?" I was dying to check his phone because I was sure he was doing something wrong! Why? Because I could do something wrong. What irritates us in others is something we do not like in ourselves! The moment I saw it – I was reborn! It seemed to relieve me! It was as if I was free. And it's not just in relationships. I get annoyed when someone is late since I started being late.

Does it annoy you that someone was messy? I've been annoyed by the mess since I got messy! Your room does not need to be cluttered to get annoyed. Maybe you are not able to tidy within. No one knows what's going on in their head, and then they get angry that the other person doesn't understand.

I remember reading what to say to get my husband to do this or that. I took courses in neurolinguistic programming and emotional intelligence with the thought that I would learn to control him. In fact, that's how I changed myself. It's funny to me now. Before, I kept silent, hid and gave replies such as "nothing," like the typical woman. And once a month I exploded! But so spectacularly! And memorably! Two to three hours of a total loss of time!

Now I have a rule – do not think more than 20 seconds. Do an experiment. Look around. Look at the woman in the store, look at the lady at the checkout, a passerby on the street – I know you will see at least one thing in an instant! Beautiful shoes! Bright color! New haircut! Say it! "Hey, you have amazing shoes!" – this is what I told the lady at the Information desk in Praktiker. "This hairstyle suits you very well!", "Your manicure is to die for!" – this, I told the lady at the bank yesterday.

And do you know what? The feeling is unique! It's like having wings! You don't walk but you fly! It is not forbidden! And the smile and emotion that is in front of you – priceless! I'm sure the person you told it to will have a completely different day! Smile at the traffic lights with the driver next to you! Completely unknown! He is confused at first, then smiles sincerely.

It's the same in the family! I used to be angry that my husband didn't understand me. Ever since I got along and started saying what I think – he understands me better! There are no ambiguities! No need to sense me! I used to say "he doesn't feel me." How could he? Is he a mind reader?!? I don't understand my own mind sometimes!

In the beginning we shared household chores. He was washing the floor, and I was angry that it wasn't washed the way I do it. He tidies around the house – but not like me! We must have had fights about this for 6 years. Then I got a maid and she had been cleaning for a few months. And guess what? Our home was perfect – clean and tidy...

But I was still dissatisfied!

Why? Because cleaning helped me relieve the stress! And I no longer had it! I stopped yelling, I stopped complaining and Ivo and I were happy! All my life I wasted time complaining about something I didn't want in the first place!

When Ivo and I met, I was wearing 12 cm heels, a short skirt, hair extensions, makeup, nails... a bimbo! It didn't matter that I was into break dancing and studying programming. I was a bimbo! I went out with boys only. I was up dancing on the bar. And guess what – **I changed**. He was very jealous. For years he wanted me to become invisible. And I did. Have you seen me with high heels? Makeup?... and guess what? He complains I look like a child now. So: **Be careful what you wish for!**

I am often asked: "He eats junk food; how can I make him stop?" Why must he eat the same things as you? You are different!

Before, I wanted to watch movies every night. I was upset he wanted a different one. He wanted to go out with friends and I wanted to read a book and have him in the house. How can he go out and I will be home alone? "Now why do you play music, it's too loud, I can't hear my thoughts from the book." Until I got it! We have different interests! Now they ask me: "Where is Ivo?" and I say "In the garage" or "I don't know" or "Out with friends." In the summer I used to be in Sveti Vlas and he was in Burgas. And reactions often were: "He has a mistress," "Aren't you jealous?" One time I remember he was out with a girl. And they call and tell me: "Ivo is with a girl in Sensa." My reaction was: "Okay." And they didn't know how to respond. Now I go to bed before 10 p.m. and there are days where I don't know what time he comes home. Despite that, I sleep very well!

When you trust yourself, you trust the other person!

There were 400 km separating us for 2 years. We went through infidelity. We went through stress news for sterility, ectopic pregnancy which was all doctors' nonsense! We went through all hormonal disbalances and crises during two pregnancies, sleep deprivation and poopy diapers. We went through our car being stolen. We lost an apartment and couldn't get it back. We lost money. We were going to hospitals, surgeries and what not! And if it wasn't all of this – it wouldn't be us! And we wouldn't be the way we are! We would turn into robots! We were only thinking about how to make money and we lost ourselves along the way! The slap afterwards was a bucket of cold water!

Health above all! Rest is a necessity and not a luxury! If you let yourself go, then you will burden the ones you love most! We should love ourselves first! We should take care of ourselves first! So, we can take care of others! We need to understand ourselves and then ask for others to understand us. People are not mind readers! We shouldn't keep it all in! It burdens only us!

In the end, everybody unwinds in their own way! First of all, you need to bring happiness to yourself! And then share it! Don't wait for the other person to make you happy! If you don't want to be happy, you will not be!

Smile! Surprise yourself! Give yourself 10 minutes for you only!

Slow down and enjoy life. Otherwise, you will not only miss what is surrounding you but you will forget where you are going and why.

Eddie Cantor

Honey ... You Are Snoring!!!

You shouldn't be pushed forward by problems but led forward by dreams.

Douglas Everette

Does this sound familiar?

When we sleep, the entire body relaxes. Muscle tone drops so that we can have effective rest and regeneration. For it to be beneficial, we need oxygen. It is responsible for the quality of thousands of processes in our body. How elastic the blood and lymph vessels are (if you do not have oxygen, varicose veins and capillaries begin to appear), determines the quality of the tissues and skin, and also determines cell regeneration and the length of your life.

Think of it as a battery attached to a charger. You can't charge it and use it at the same time.

Have you ever got up in the morning and felt like you haven't gone to bed? Well, then you used it, not charged it!

When we snore, the body does not have enough oxygen. Instead of resting, you make it work to make up for that lack.

Why do we actually snore and how to get rid of it?

I really like it when somebody says to me: "I snore because I sleep on my back"! This is the most accurate sleeping position! This is not the reason! It is amazing that there are even "healing ways" how not to sleep on your back invented. From a ball that has thorns and is sewn to our pajamas on our chests and backs to teach us to sleep on one side to those that vibrate, squeak, electrocute etc.

1. Excessive weight – the accumulation of adipose tissue is like training for 24 hours with weights from 2 to 80 kg. There is no time to rest. The muscles are in constant spasm or at the other extreme – they give up, like their owner. In the supine position, adipose tissue compresses the airways. Imagine a straw, but you squeeze it with two fingers, the juice passes but with difficulty. And now squeeze it with your whole hand... is something passing through? Not very satisfying, is it? Separately, all these excess fat sacs compress the blood and lymph vessels, the muscles do not feed, do not clean and become a dump. But we have already talked about that. Here, as a start, we need to lose weight.

2. Relaxed muscles – everyone knows that you need to train for a shredded back, for a healthy waist, for a tight ass, for a flat stomach. And how many of you train your face? The muscles of the face depend on each other. Imagine a puzzle. Each part depends on the others to stay in place. We start from the forehead, then the eye contour, followed by the nose, cheeks, cheekbones, lips, tongue, chin, neck. When we sleep, the tongue falls down to the throat. An indication that it is relaxed is a light double chin. The neck, on the other hand, if it has the "Venus Ring" wrinkles as if it has one, two or three necklaces around the neck, and they do not have to be deep, means that we have weakness in the neck. The solution is a workout for the facial muscles – Face building or another type.

3. We breathe shallowly – if we breathe incorrectly in our daily life, we breathe the same way in our sleep. We breathe shallowly, we use the lungs only in their upper part. The solution is diaphragm training. It is done with an elastic band, in a very specific position and certain

sensations are sought – burning between the ribs, pain in the vertebrae on the back at the level of the bra, etc.

4. Chronic distortions in the nostrils and narrowed space – here only surgery comes to the rescue.

5. Cold, sinusitis, bacterial infection – over 50% of people on the planet do not even know about candida, bacteria and infections, living in them. In addition to mucus, which is harmful for us, they also cause many health problems. It is easiest to go and give sputum, nasal and throat secretions. Thus, if the laboratory is capable, it will certainly find the presence of a fungus or bacterium in at least one place. In this case, either take an antibiotic prescribed by a doctor on an antibiogram, or some natural remedies. For example, the last time the children caught Moraxela, we were cured with a very strong tea from a Russian healer. What we eat is also very important here – no fast carbohydrates and sugars, alcohol, etc. Each bacterium is sensitive to certain herbs and feeds on sweets.

6. Infection of the tonsils and adenoids (glands between the nose and throat, slightly smaller than the tonsils). When inflamed, they swell and narrow the airways.

7. Alcohol – enhances muscle relaxation. The respiratory muscles, diaphragm and liver work thanks to their muscles. If we let the muscles go you can already guess what's going on. The solution is not to drink before bed.

8. Spinal curvature – causes pressure and blockages, raises the pressure in the chest. The solution is corrective gymnastics. The condition of the muscular and skeletal structure is determined. Each joint is checked – how much it is displaced and twisted. You say what else you want to achieve – tightening, losing weight, shredding or something else. How much time do you have and where do you want to train – gym, at home? You have

to combine it all. If you're wondering how I know – my brother does just that. He showed me how, what and why and thanks to him we created SEMMA. Write "Kristiyan Belchev" or enter the website and you will see a lot of useful information on the subject.

9. Pillow – it compresses important arteries, slows down metabolic processes, distorts the cervical spine and compresses the airways. The solution – sleep on your back without a pillow.

10. Some medications – the intake of magnesium in large quantities, as well as some other medications and supplements, cause muscle relaxation.

11. Pregnancy – the baby grows, the lungs and all organs climb up to the diaphragm. Everything is very tight and cramped. We start breathing very shallowly. The solution here is to try to breathe as properly as possible in our daily lives by opening the diaphragm to the side. This way we will also have prevention against varicose veins! The magnesium, which we are prescribed in addition, relaxes the muscles. It is good to sleep on one side with your back straight, not as a fetus. The legs should not be bent, but stretched forward diagonally without distorting the waist. In the early months, it helps to sleep on your back with your arms raised above your head. This opens the chest.

Snoring is not a problem! It is an indication that something is wrong and a problem will occur! It's like the red light on the dashboard. If you are a woman, you have no idea what it means. You go to someone and tell them, "A red light is on, come and check it" because you know that if it stays on, your car may leave you somewhere along the way! Snoring is an oxygen deficiency! An oxygen deficiency equals fast aging and atrophy of tissues, muscles and organs, poor memory, varicose veins, weight gain, low sensitivity, heart problems (heart attack, stroke) and any disease that is currently going through your head. Start snoring, or vice versa, think about when the light came on, and don't excuse yourself with the phrase, "I've been snoring for 15 years." People living with you are not to blame! You are the only person who has a real benefit to do something for yourself – **Now!**

For every minute you are angry you lose sixty seconds of happiness.

Ralph Waldo Emerson

Wrinkles

The secret of a happy life is enjoying small things every day.

William Morris

Skin problems are not to be underestimated. We don't talk about esthetics and beauty but health!

When we see a wrinkle the reaction is: "It's the aging, it's normal!" Wrinkles are a factor in the aging process – yes. But we do not age only in the skin. Wrinkles on the outside show that the regeneration process is slowed down! Regeneration in tissues and organs is delayed!

Yes — this means that at the present moment your life is shortening!

Don't you want to live for at least 120 years?

Imagine the skin as the dashboard of a car. There are thousands of lights that show you the problem before it gets hot and the car stops. Now I will teach you how to read the lights on your skin.

1. Wrinkles – breakdown of collagen fibers! Low quality collagen! If the maximum quality is 100%, then in the case of improper nutrition the collagen fibers break down and at the same time their quality drops to 20–30–40%. The main layer of the skin is 80% collagen, the joints are 70% collagen, the bones are 30% collagen. With proper development, the protein in our body is from 40 to 60%. Thirty percent of it is collagen. Roughly speaking, 15 and 20% of our entire body is collagen.
2. Skin sagging – lack of protein in the diet! Protein is 30% collagen!

3. Pimples – a body infection. Different products cause different infections – pimples with white tips, subcutaneous, blackheads. It is very important how long after that the scar remains, where the pimple is and the like. Sugar, dairy products, gluten, white salt, alcohol — each of these products may cause infections in muscles and tissues. To protect itself, the body encapsulates them with fat cells and retracts them for further processing. This way it prevents complete toxicity and breakdown in the body. The bud on the outside shows the condition on the inside. Therefore, we do not need to apply 1000 creams against skin infections, but to think about the cause. Because we shower with medicines, creams and makeup, we have no idea what we look like from the inside. From a suppressed childhood rash on the skin, the infection turns inward even more and kills the lungs, and from there appears Asthma (these are the words of the grandson of a Russian healer who received one of the four prizes "Contribution to Russia").

4. Smelly sweat – a sign that we are toxic! And all these ointments, which stop sweating at this point, stop the body from removing toxins and poison. It has no other way to get rid of rubbish except through sweat, urine, feces!

5. Facial color pale yellow – lack of vitamin C (from 600 to 1000 mg per day). Responsible for the quality, color and elasticity of the skin.

If the face is dull and matt, we have a problem with skin, hair, nails, weight gain, acne, overeating, heart pain – it lacks sulfur (you can find it in onions, broccoli, parsley, apples, arugula, cabbage, soy, barley, bee pollen).

Wrinkles, stretch marks, rosacea, pigmentation, hair loss are a sign of zinc deficiency. It is contained in seeds, algae, spinach, coconut, spirulina. Helps to form new collagen.

Wrinkles also appear in the absence of silicon. It is a major link in joints, bones, cartilage, connective tissue and collagen. You can find it in nettle, oats, cucumbers, greens.

Vitamin D + calcium + magnesium – responsible for quality, color, elasticity of the skin. There is a perfect combination in sesame and almonds. If we take calcium without vitamin D, we do not absorb it. The lack of magnesium is observed if we have muscle cramps in the evening.

B vitamins – in their absence the skin has no elasticity. It looks sluggish and tired. The problem is not the skin, but it shows us that we will soon have a problem with the nervous system. In the absence of vitamin B, we are nervous, irritable and crooked. We produce a lot of stress and enter storage mode.

If our skin is flabby, slightly gray or greenish, or we are constantly cold, our body tells us that we are deficient in iron. It must be taken with vitamin C. I eat nettle to get it.

If we want cleaner, lighter skin, then we need vitamins E and A – these are antioxidants that are responsible for skin color. Poor skin color means that the body cannot detoxify. And at the present moment we are poisoned. The best option is to mix vitamins A, E and C. Each increases the influence of the other two.

If you have dehydrated skin – the first dehydration begins in the bone marrow. Only then are we thirsty. To get to the skin, the situation is serious! We suffer from poor memory, we have pain in the back and spine, we begin to hunch over as the intersegmental liquid is 80% water. The spine loses density and problems such as scoliosis, kyphosis and the like begin.

Oily skin – excessive secretion of sebaceous glands! It is a rarity! More often, dry skin, to compensate for its dryness, begins to produce a lot of sebum in a short time. This is from dehydration or flushing.

Pigmentation – most often from gluten and allergy to it.

Bags and dark circles – weakness in the muscles of the eye area. This is an indicator of muscle weakness, responsible for the movement and functioning of the eyes. If you work on this muscle with exercises, diopters and future diseases of the eyes are removed. These two problems are an indication of muscle weakness and fluid retention. The body does not swell in one place! It swells everywhere, we just don't see it. Swelling under the eyes also means swelling in the brain.

Swelling in the face – a problem with the circulation of lymph and blood. The lymph cleans the garbage and unnecessary substances. When it is not working it is like not passing a garbage truck. It's okay for a day, it's okay for two, and in two weeks? The blood carries nutrients. How will you feel without food for two weeks?

Next time, think before you decide it's just another pimple!

Do not take supplements to get collagen. First, stop eating food that breaks it down. And then intensify its synthesis! It's like building something on foundations that you know will fall.

Many people miss happiness not because they didn't find it, but because they didn't take a break to enjoy it.

William Feather

What Is a Metabolic Type?

Let's go back to when there were no planes and cars. People born in the cold live their whole lives in the cold. Those born in the sun live their entire lives in the sun.

What is happening?

It's cold! No greens, only ice and big game (protein and fat). To absorb protein from meat, we need about 4 hours. The stomach is a muscle that can tighten and relax. Thanks to this and the acids, it crushes food. That's why it's good to chew, because our stomach doesn't have teeth. I'm sure everyone remembers someone who swallows like a "fit." The stomach has no teeth! It needs mushy food to further process. Not chunks. The stomach pushes the smoothie to the intestines and there begins the great assimilation. Imagine the intestines as suction cups. They suck up the liquid and leave the solid to pass through the feces, so the protein types have about 7 meters from the mouth to the anus, they have more concentrated gastric juices, they are often hungry and nervous if they do not eat.

Second case – it's warm! Africa, tropics... Lots of greens, fruits, vegetables (fiber and carbohydrates). Protein is the main building block in everyone's diet. The difference is how we will get it and from what. Vegetable protein is bound to fiber. It takes a very long fermentation to digest. These people have 14 meter-long digestive systems from mouth to anus. They digest more slowly and need about 6 hours until the next meal. Why is that? Because it takes more time to extract plant protein.

How is this actually proven? Dr. Byron Robinson performed 650 dissections on humans. He proved that individuals living in the north (winter and cold) have a 7-meter digestive system. This is a protein type (polar). People living on the equator (summer and heat) have a 14-meter digestive system. This is a carbohydrate type (equatorial). And in a place with a temperate climate (all seasons) are found mixed types – from 7 to 14 meters.

That's why there are so many diets. That's why they work for one and not for another.

That's why I'm firmly against all diets! Everyone loses weight differently. You are very unlikely to come across your diet. And to find it, it takes a lot of experience, stress and time. The easiest way is to learn how food affects your emotions and the condition of your body. To find where you are on the scale of light – heavy protein/unsaturated – saturated carbohydrate/light – heavy fat. And then move up and down the scale depending on your daily routine (mental and physical exertion, stress, period, etc.). In three months, everything becomes a habit. You learn to understand your body and don't even think about what and why you eat.

Recall the example of the dog and Pavlov's lamp. The lamp clicks, food is given. One time, second, third, fifth... fiftieth... The lamp clicks, the dog comes, saliva flows, food – no. So is the body. Today you have no energy – the body wants chocolate or coffee. You are sad – the body wants sugar and white flour. If you give it something else for one month, in a month it will want the other. You have no energy – you will eat greasy food. It could be nuts, it could be bacon, it could be butter or something. It depends on what type you are.

In one family, everyone is a different type. That is why separate cooking is good. So, one will have more meat, another will eat only vegetables, a third will want mixed. I eat very greasy and heavy, my little daughter is close to me, and the eldest only wants fruits and vegetables. My husband, on the other hand, wants something radically different. I eat bacon, the older one – butter. Our breakfast: Aliya – hearts, bacon, banana. Me – eggs, tomato, butter. Ivayla – smoothie made of apple, walnuts, flaxseed, sunflower, fresh thyme, etc. Ivo eats an omelet. Dinner: Me – sunflower, pumpkin seeds and butter soup, Aliya – steak with butter, Iva – roasted broccoli, red beets, Ivo – steak with tomatoes. We enjoy eating what we need. What tastes good to us may be awful to others.

I love it when someone tells me:

"For the first time in my life I eat what I want and lose weight."

Bad conscience, bad combination and stereotypes are what hinder us. Everything is embedded in our genes, and new technologies dull our senses. We have forgotten our own language. That of our body. Everyone who has a pet knows that when a dog has a stomach ache, it eats grass. And it is precisely defined which grass. Hardly his mother taught him what kind of grass would be in our garden.

The best diet is the one that is for you! One that does not deprive you, but helps you build a habit! The one that makes you happy!

If you are wondering what I'm talking about – go to our website. In the Free category, at the request of my customers, I have uploaded examples of my foods. I am mixed to protein type. The idea is not to copy them, but to see how many different combinations you can make. My goal is to break your understanding of food.

Be different! Be yourself!

Keep smiling, because life is a beautiful thing and there's so much to smile about.

Marylin Monroe

How We Can Eat Less and Enjoy More!

We've all studied taste buds in biology class but do we remember it? We usually eat something in a hurry. The portion is eaten in seconds, and if it's something sweet, we don't even feel like we've eaten it. Not to mention then how heavy we feel after. We wonder who made us eat all that.

Well, there is a solution

Look at the picture and remember it. You have four zones. And depending on what you eat, you chew in that area. Keep the food there and you will feel real enjoyment of what you eat. So, you do not need to eat 2 bars of chocolates, cake and what not. The sweet is only on the tip of the tongue! When was the last time you kept a sweet bite at the tip of your tongue? Hardly. We live in a hurry and forget about the little pleasures! Do not deprive yourself of them! When the taste is saturated, then we are saturated with better quality without wanting more.

If you like the idea, share it with friends. Don't be stingy.

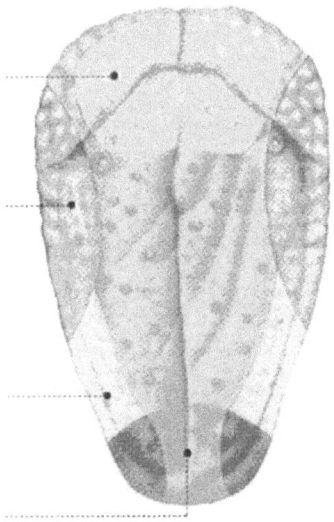

Desires must be fulfilled right away. Otherwise, you lose the pleasure. If you want something – do it, life is short. Here and now!

Michal Weller

Sugar Continued

If you don't like what you get, change what you give.

Carlos Castaneda

Remember that pastry shop I told you about? All those people who were looking for "something sweet"? They were overweight. Wide pelvis and thighs. A boy came in, around third grade. He was short and very chubby. He said, "One of these," with such sadness that it made me get goosebumps! He hadn't eaten the sweets yet but he was already feeling guilty! I couldn't wait to be given the saucer with the little fork.

Then a family came in: a mother, a father and two approximately 16-year-old girls. Excess weight, acne of all kinds (white small pimples on the forehead – caused by dairy products, acne foci in 5–6 places on the face, dark pigmentation from unhealed pimples – from sugar and gluten). They had a strong asymmetry. The father was so happy and asked everyone if they wanted two pieces of cake. Why not only one? I'm writing it now and I'm sad. The mother was about 45 years old. And she had not escaped the effect. Her face was like that of a teenager in puberty. And they were not happy. The three women were angry that they would eat it. The dad was happy to make them smile.

How does sugar affect you?

I will allow myself to steal a description written by my brother in his textbook:

100 years ago, the average consumption was about 1.8 kg of sugar per year per capita on the planet. In 2015, a study was conducted in England and it was seen that consumption increased to 68–77 kg per person per

year. In Bulgaria it is 36 kg. Pyruvic acid accumulates in the brain, nervous system and red blood cells. This ingredient interferes with cell respiration. The cells are suffocating. It's like putting a plastic bag on your head. So, the cell dies. And it is the beginning of degenerative diseases. Sugar also leads to an acidic state, which extracts minerals from teeth and bones in the body's attempt to alkalize again. High blood sugar stimulates the release of insulin to lower it. The feedback is slow and we fall into a state of low blood sugar. This stimulates the production of the stress hormone cortisol. It causes us to release the hidden glycogen from the liver to raise blood sugar. And so, some people live in this cycle – low – high blood sugar. The diseases caused are of all types, such as a tendency to violence, anger, nervousness, cancer, schizophrenia, inability to concentrate, problems with teeth and organs.

Artificial sweeteners are not a better solution. Aspartame has received more complaints of side effects than any other dietary supplement in history. These sweeteners trick our body into thinking we are giving it sweets, which means nutrients. When the substances reach our intestines, the body finds that it does not receive them and makes us continue to eat. Some artificial sweeteners can also damage our nervous system.

In other words, white refined sugar raises our blood sugar. From there we release insulin, followed by cortisol. After 20–30 minutes we are hungry again and we want another dose. We raise it again, it drops again. As a **bonus**, we enter the "stockpile" mode. If we have stress hormones, we do not use but preserve them.

Second bonus – we cause infection throughout the body – tissues and organs. In order not to infect the whole body, it encapsulates the harmful substances in fat bubbles and stores it for later. Only, this "later" never comes!

What about the squeezes that everyone loves? Let's take 4 apples. If they are whole, we will eat 1–2, the fiber will saturate us and we will say "enough." If we make them into juice, however, the fiber is gone. Vitamins and fructose remain. We can drink much more than 2 apples from the juice. An apple has about 4 teaspoons of sugar, and here are 16 teaspoons of sugar in a cup. You don't have to eat junk food to eat too much sugar, and cause internal obesity.

Vitamin waters have approximately 5 teaspoons of sugar, green tea – 8.5 teaspoons. All drinks have between 5 and 15 tsp. at 600 ml. With this mode of 40 tsp. per day for 12 days we will gain about 4 kg. And here the problem is not that we have gained weight. All this is internal fat located between our organs. It pressures and interferes with their work. Can you think of anyone with a belly? Well, it's internal fat. This type of gaining weight is followed by many metabolic diseases, heart disease, type 2 diabetes.

When we eat a lot of sugar and other carbohydrates, we take in a lot of glucose and fructose. The body begins to secrete insulin. It captures glucose and we do not burn it as energy. What's the catch? As long as we have insulin, we store fat. And so, we release insulin to process fructose. At this point, we cannot use the fat made from fructose, but store it. Thus, there is no way to have a high level of fructose in the blood and at the same time to process glucose.

Motivation is always more important than mere talent.
Norman Augustin

SOS!!! Oily Skin!!! SOS!!!

Today I got up at 04:00 and thought about a thing related to the skin that I repeat every day. I wanted to write something that would be super useful for you! Then I remembered the nightmares I had during the summer evenings. How I kept repeating the same thing, and the ignorant were always around! I worked as a beautician for over 12 hours a day in my parlors and worked in two at the same time. Between 15 and 25 people passed through my hands a day. I repeated more than 10 times a day: "Your skin is not oily, but dehydrated, because..." And how many times have I repeated it in my sleep? This is another topic!

Today, many people do not really realize what oily skin is and what is dehydrated! Why does this happen? In both cases, the skin becomes oily and has enlarged pores and blackheads. The forehead shines and whatever we put on, we want to wash or wipe it off in 5 minutes. We wash our face in the morning and in the evening, apply light creams or skip them altogether. Are you familiar with this?

What do we do? We've been out all day, at work, soaking up the dust from the streets. We have a layer of sebum, a layer of cream, a layer of makeup and finally a few layers of dust and garbage. We go home and take a wonderful warm shower, if possible hot. It dissolves fat formations; the heat dehydrates the skin as a bonus. Then we come out of the shower and don't want to put anything on our skin, perhaps just a very light cream. In the morning we get up and feel that the face is oily and wash it again. We can put on cream again. Makeup on top. And we wonder why we are greasy; we constantly touch our face or stick rubbish to it. Ah, here! A pimple also appeared.

If we wash the skin in the morning, we remove its protection (the sebum, which it has been diligently producing all night).

The body is very smart. It knows what protection it will need the next day. And it produces it! If we wash it in the morning and go outside after 15 minutes, we are unprotected. Panicked skin begins to produce the same amount of sebum, but not for 8–10 hours of sleep, but for 15 minutes. The body is not stupid. It works in sync. If you give it 15 minutes from washing to exposure, it will learn. But if you have to produce 1 tsp. sebum in 12 hours, so you will produce it in 15 minutes. Your face shines and your skin is dry. Think of it as an order. If you order 10 buns (let's say they are healthy) for after 12 hours, but you burn the portion by reheating it a little before they come, you will make new ones, right? But this time you will be more expeditious! You will not say: "Well, so what, I will give them a refund of two thousand leva."

Stop living for what is behind the corner and start enjoying the walk on the street.

Grand Miller

Why does the face get greasy? What is sebum? Imagine that this is the cream of your skin. It makes a protective film every day, and its release is influenced by your hormones, your daily life, stress and external factors – environment (wind, sun, cold, heat...).

The second reason is creams, detergents and cosmetics. If they have SLS, mineral oil, parabens, Vaseline, antifreeze (propylene glycol), paraffin, glycerin, phthalates, placenta and the like, then you have a greenhouse effect. If you put gloves on your hands and you wear them non-stop, what will happen in a week? What about in two, three .. two months...?! It's the same with these products. They make a greenhouse effect – stretch film over the skin. The skin sweats, loses water. At the same time, the skin sensors say it is dry and it produces sebum. The pores become enlarged – on the one hand, so that the sebum comes out faster, on the other – because it is a greenhouse. All the rubbish goes deeper, inflammation and permanent blackheads begin. **The solution: wash your face only in the evening!**

If you use micellar water – then wash with water! We will soon talk about the difference between thermal and micellar waters. Then we apply a cream that makes us feel wonderful in the morning! The skin should not be oily, it should not be dry. If one day your cream is okay, it does not mean that it will be every day. Just as you want a salad one day and then a greasy steak, so does your skin. Don't put anything on your face that you wouldn't eat! We take many times more substances through the skin than through the mouth. Use clean products. With 1 to 6 ingredients. These creams have a shelf life of 6 months to one year.

So, wash the face only once. We use cream for today! We have three creams – light, oily and serum. And we combine them differently according to the needs of our skin! Listen to it! It loves to show what is wrong with it. If it is oily, drink more water, smear with lemon and wash after 20 minutes before the evening cream. You can make a mask with protein and lemon again in 20 minutes. You can use natural collagen. If you are over 30 years old – use hyaluronic acid as well. Yogurt – if not from the store. Half a piece of brewer's yeast with water again for 20 minutes. We can spread some fruit or vegetable as well and stay like this for 20 minutes.

But above all, stop drying it with cosmetics and washing! Every skin is different and it is different even from yesterday's self. Give it 7 days to change completely. If you stop torturing it, you will see how it will become your best friend in 7 days!

Today do what others don't want to and tomorrow you will live like others can't.

Jared Leto

Are You Nervous? Is Everything Irritating You?

There is only one way to do a lot of work – to love what you do.

Steve Jobs

You are lacking B Vitamins

You, however, should be very careful with this one. Years ago, I used to drink brewer's yeast. Do you remember? When you have acne a lot of doctors used to prescribe it. Why?

Because it contains folic acid. It affects DNA division and the formation of new cells. It increases the ability to accelerate its recovery. If you usually manage to repair 10% of the damage, then with it you manage 40%, etc. Folic acid "repairs" the cell from the inside out!

Over the centuries, queens, empresses, "khaleesi" – all had given birth at the age of 40! When we are pregnant and we eat properly the body regenerates. We feed the fetus, and it feeds us. We help it create stem cells to build itself. It gives us stem cells to rebuild us. That's how everyone wins. That's why I get very annoyed when someone tells me, "I'm pregnant, pregnancy screwed me." You screw yourself!

But back to the topic. Folic acid is very important. Next is magnesium. It relaxes! It is no coincidence that when you have muscle cramps, they always tell you that you don't take enough magnesium. For what has been said so far, I use Nutritional Yeast. There are many different ones in organic stores and on the Internet. They have fibers, copper, zinc, sodium, iron. But it's mainly B vitamins.

You can again find it in organic stores. Do you remember the big trees in Africa – baobab. I also add baobab dust. It contains more vitamin C than lemon. Do you remember the deep wrinkles article? The skin radiates after a baobab mask because it contains potassium, calcium, iron, manganese, sodium, phosphorus, zinc, vitamins A, B1, B2, B3, B6.

To finish, I add ginkgo biloba powder. This tree lives for over 1,000 years. And there is a reason.

And now I will give you the overall picture from afar. We have folic acid. I enhance the production in the cell factory. From there we have vitamins A and C – strong antioxidants. We throw out the rubbish. We give iron, potassium, calcium, phosphorus, magnesium, sodium – building blocks of trace elements. First, we increase the production and the second time, we give building materials. Magnesium and B vitamins calm the nervous system. So first we clean, then we build. But for all this to happen, our blood vessels must be open. Ginkgo biloba and baobab have the ability to do so. Why is ginkgo biloba in every pill for memory? Because it improves the flow of oxygen. There is oxygen, there is energy, there is regeneration. The combination itself is unique. And the strangest thing is that no one selling supplements has made a package for this!

Many people drink supplements, but they do not get where they need to. Because the circulatory system and lymph flow are blocked. First unclog the channel, strengthen the pipes and then put in the useful substances!

Try it and feel how calm you will be. Nobody cares that you get angry. You decide whether to get on your nerves or not! Being angry means producing stress hormones. It means entering the weight gain mode. It means you can't regenerate. It means aging artificially! Think about whether it's worth shortening your life by a year because of an idiot who crossed your path, for example. Because someone pushed you and spilled your coffee. That the child has spilled water on the new sofa or drew on the wall. Look for the fun, look for the joy.

If, after all, someone has made you angry and you lose your temper, you have my number! I will help you cleanse.

Have a nice day, Fairy!

You will fail. You will get hurt. You will make mistakes. You will have periods of depression and despair. Family, education, work, everyday problems – all of it can hinder your training. Despite, your inner compass should always point in one direction – the goal.

Stuart McRobert

Oxygen

Did you notice that many of the pages revolve around oxygen? We mentioned it at least once. Nowadays we are so in a hurry to go somewhere, that we are even out of breath. We forget how good it is to breathe! I often say in trainings: "Stop breathing and you will be relieved!"

We breathe so shallowly that we get a minimum satisfactory percentage of oxygen, just enough to exist! What are we? Why should we live with so little! We keep complaining that someone is depriving us of this and that! And in fact, we deprive ourselves?

We've already talked about it — only cancer cells live without oxygen!

Oxygen = Energy!

Have you noticed how when it was cold, you end the long working day, you are tired, you have no strength, you go out and you take a deep breath. And everything changes! It's as if something fills you from within at the same moment. And if it could be like that every day! 24 hours a day!

Studies on chlamydia (bacteria that are sexually transmitted and lead to infertility) have shown that the immune system can only fight them if there is enough oxygen in the lining of the vagina. If there is not enough oxygen, chlamydia multiplies rapidly and inflammation occurs. The same happens with Helicobacter pylori, as well as with bacteria that cause heart attacks and strokes. These are bacteria that must be treated with antibiotics!

When we smoke, carbon monoxide is released. It binds to hemoglobin in the blood, which transports oxygen from the lungs to the tissues. Respectively – prevent and delay!

We will soon talk about acidity and alkalinity. We are acidic in the absence of oxygen. Excessive amounts of meat, pastries, dairy and the like cause high acidity in the connective tissue. This makes it difficult for oxygen and nutrients to reach the cells. Something like a traffic jam at the end of the working day in Sofia.

What does oxygen do? Gives cells energy. It occurs in the mitochondria, their power plants. If there is not enough oxygen, the brain, organs, muscles and nerves do not work normally.

Today, everyone is crazy about oxygen therapies. Oxygen has been everywhere for several years now. In cosmetics each brand has a therapy to saturate the skin with oxygen. There are three therapies in medicine. Ozone therapy – in it, patients first receive a cocktail of vitamins and minerals. It improves the uptake of oxygen into the cells. They then inhale oxygen-enriched air. There are therapies with intravenous infusion. There are also pressure chambers. Used before for diver training. And it all costs a solid amount of money. And a bonus: it's not done once! You do it —you have a result; you stop and little by little you return to the start.

By inhaling the air, it enters the pulmonary alveoli. Imagine it as many streets connected. Where the street ends as a dead end is in the form of a bubble. This bubble is the alveolus. Hemoglobin, produced by red blood cells, binds to oxygen. The protein molecules then bind to them and carry it through the bloodstream into the arteries and blood vessels. An exchange takes place in the capillaries. Oxygen is replaced with the carbon dioxide from the muscle. Pure barter. The garbage returns to the lung and we exhale.

When muscles work, they produce a lot of carbon dioxide and lactic acid. These are waste products. They are cleaned with oxygen. If you get tired during training, and then you have sore muscles – you are not breathing!

The "I need oxygen" alert comes after you are already in deficit!

The diaphragm can be shortened once. Either inhale or exhale. You choose! If you emphasize exhalation – you fall into deficit. It tightens, expels oxygen and relaxes when inhaled. You inhale a little and shallowly. If you tighten on inhalation, you inhale a lot of oxygen. And you relax on the exhale. That way you don't exhale to the end. There is a reserve of oxygen until the next inhalation.

From hunching the back and lack of training for the diaphragm, it weakens. We crush the liver and breathe shallowly. We are satisfied with nuts! What is diaphragm training – breathing! In our "Stand Yourself Up in 6 Weeks" campaign, uploaded on our website, we showed you an exercise about this in Video 1! If you haven't done it already – do it!

A strong diaphragm equals a strong center! You will be upright! You will be healthy! Your cells will work like a 20-year-old individual! If you are 40 years old, this is half your life! If you are 60 years old – this is half of your conscious life!

Half the people wear waist belts when training because they have a weak core! The real belt is our lower abdominal wall, waist and diaphragm!

We do not need expensive breathing procedures! This is another trick of the industry to make us slaves to the grave!

Learn to breathe. Sit down! Straighten your back! Look ahead! Inhale 30 times fast. Emphasize this on inhalation! And on the exhale just open your mouth. Inhale 30 times, exhale and hold without air. When you think you can't do it anymore, hold for another 20 seconds. Now inhale and hold for 10 seconds with oxygen in the lungs! Are you dizzy?!? Here is oxygen! This is a method by which I have treated the symptoms of asthma, varicose veins and other diseases!

Everyone who comes to SEMMA knows how they get dizzy when breathing! Enjoy!

Smile all day, Lovely one! Breathe!

When you have difficulties, you shouldn't give up and run. Assess the situation so you can seek a solution and believe that everything happens for the better. Patience is the key to victory.

Nick Vujicic

SLS?!? What the Hell Is That?

This is the foaming agent in every product. Ninety-eight to one hundred percent of our shampoos, shower gels, liquid soaps and face cleansers, creams, body oils, toothpastes, household products and what not, contain it!

SLS has different variations – sodium lauryl (laurel) sulfate (sodium lauryl sulfate) or sodium lauryl sulfate. Other names are: sodium dodecyl sulphate, sodium PEG lauryl sulphate, monododecyl ester, sodium PEG lauryl ether sulphate This product is from oil refining, which is often masked with the inscription "derived from coconut oil" or "from coconuts," ammonium lauryl sulfate – ALS and ammonium lauryl sulfate – ALES, sodium lauryl sulfate (SLES) and many more.

And before I lose your interest, I'll just stop listing. Many variations – one goal, one product.

The problem is that these substances are one of the most concentrated in the products described above. The content on the label is arranged from the most saturated ingredients in the product to the least contained. And they are always among the top 2 or 5 of the content.

SLS is used in many clinics around the world to induce skin irritation in experimental subjects. The researchers then remove the irritation of the damaged areas of the skin with various preparations, analyzing their effectiveness.

Since the birth of my children, there has been nothing at home with SLS. SLS was added to the soap we used about a year ago. The reaction on my eldest daughter's hands was peeling and the onset of dermatitis. When I used SLS shampoos, I washed my hair every other day! It was unthinkable to wash it once every 5 days. I had oily roots and constantly had split ends. Now I train every day and wash my hair once every 5 days! And for the last 7 months, my hair has not had a single split end without being cut.

It is also found in anti-dandruff shampoos. It makes a film like stretch film and seals dandruff beneath it. So, while we wash, we don't see the white particles and we think we've dealt with the problem. The next time we wash, together with the foam, we remove this film, and with it the scales from the scalp. And then we seal again. The seal is not always 100% and sometimes there is still slight dandruff. If we stop using the shampoo, the dandruff intensifies because we have suffocated the scalp.

I will now give you an excerpt from the research of the Medical College of the University of Georgia:

SLS cleans by oxidizing the surface. In other words, it makes it unprotected against bacteria. Kills its natural protective layer – the alkaline. And for the cover makes a greenhouse effect, leaving a stop – layer. The skin becomes dehydrated and bacteria, candida and infections begin to develop in the bag. Irritating to skin, causing itching, flaking, redness, allergies and long-term skin diseases.

Thanks to the greenhouse effect, SLS dries the hair, causes the formation of dry, breakable and blooming tips, can contribute to hair loss and dandruff, as well as diseases of the scalp.

SLS makes hair greasy at the roots, causing the need to wash your head much more often. Everything is very simple – the strong degreasing of the scalp stimulates the active work of the sebaceous glands. Furthermore, SLS was made up during World War II to wash oil and rust off of tanks.

SLS penetrates through the skin into tissues and organs, including the eyes, liver, kidneys, heart, brain, stays there and accumulates gradually, increasing its concentration. SLS can change the protein composition of cells, especially in children, causing various diseases, for example, cataracts. It causes cell mutations and can damage the immune system.

Sulfates react with many of the components in cosmetics, forming nitrosamines (nitrates) and carcinogenic dioxins. They also penetrate the skin and then the blood.

It is not excreted by the liver, but accumulates in the body!

Mainly causes cancer! It prevents oxygen from entering the cell. And we've already said – the only cell that exists without oxygen is the cancer cell. In reality, our body adapts to our way of life. Cancer is not a disease! Cancer is a mutation! Which you cause yourself!

And now I know your brain says, "I need to detox, clean it up!"

Don't ponder on how to clean it up! Stop using it!

I can give you a thousand names of universities that have done research, but they are unlikely to convince you. I'll just lose you in the lines and you will move on.

Unfortunately, the inscriptions on the bottle "suitable for children," "approved for children's use," do not guarantee the absence of these harmful and dangerous substances.

There are two options to produce a product – pure, expensive, without foam, which people do not like. It will be appreciated by very few who value their health. Or cheap, foaming, liked by people, bought by everybody?!? Tough choice, isn't it?

When entering an organic store and reading the packaging, I would not buy more than 60% of what is offered. When it says "vegan," "organic," "for children" it is complete nonsense! A trade trick to sell. It takes you several years to get inside of things. Even when I want to buy something, I stand at the store, open the site www.ewg.org/skindeep and check every single ingredient I don't know! And only then will I buy. That's why I hate to change a product. If I find something I'm happy with –

it's it! I tell it "yes" until the suspension of the production or if modification separates us!

I am wishing you an unforgettable and fresh day!

Let it be as great as you are!

All the art of living lies in a fine mingling of letting go and holding on.

Havelock Ellis

How Much Do You Cost?

Failure is just an opportunity to start over, but wiser.

Henry Ford

Some facts over the past 10 years!

Do you love yourself? How much? How much do you think your health costs? How much are you willing to pay and give to be healthy? And for your children to be healthy? And the ones you love?

Let me tell you something.

I did anti-cellulite procedures for 8 years. I explained to each woman how to eat, what cosmetics to use, posture, breathing, water, what not to do, etc. We usually had packages of 10 procedures of 1 hour each. I had 10 hours to change their lives! But when I got to the part with sports, with movement and how to keep the result, the answer was: "I prefer to come at 6 months and not have to think about it!" They preferred to give 1,600 leva, but not to move!!!

In the beauty parlor I did basically two things: acne therapies and anti-aging procedures! People wanted to either get rid of their wrinkles or get rid of acne. I talked about both things, what causes them, why they exist. What do they mean? How wrinkles are her least problem! The real enemy is the breakdown of collagen in the body! It really falls apart from the inside out! I explain how she should not take a thousand collagen tablets, but stop taking the products that cause it to break down.

With acne I give examples, I nag, I talk... How is it a problem and an infection in the lipid layer, in the lymph, in the disposal of toxins. That they should not treat the consequence, but the real cause. You really need to stop taking substances that cause the infection and then the face will just glow!

It's the same with swelling. We do not fight the swelling, but we fight the food and the habit that causes it.

And most people's responses were, "I'd rather come here in 30 days so you can make me smooth again and not deal with nonsense." "Well, I'm not going to live 100 years, I'm 40 now." "I've been battling acne my whole life, let's burn it, will I clean it now?" "My mom was dealing with swelling a lot, it's genetic..."

At festivals, to which we were invited to the big malls, people were constantly repeating the excuse **"I have no time,"** and they were wasting 5–7 hours walking between two floors! Everyone stopped for the prizes, because each was worth 260 leva. Until they realized that the prizes were two training cards that would straighten their spine, teach them to breathe, etc. At that moment, we lost them, everyone wants a magic pill, not to put in effort.

For the last 3 months I have been invited to be a lecturer in over 20 cities. And by people who have already made a name for themselves! We had to have over 20 Masterclasses. And do you know? Half dropped out with the words: "I do not understand! This is for health and there is no interest! If it was for some nonsense and money, they would find time!" Why? Because everyone chooses the easy way! Everyone chooses to close their eyes to their true condition. Everyone compares himself to the people he sees. Everyone is like blind horses! You go out and all your peers are just like you! There is no longer an adequate basis for comparison! And the one that is left is considered the elite – these are people with a lot of money, don't look at them! They live well!

A healthy lifestyle is not that expensive! Being upright doesn't cost money! Breathe properly too – oxygen is free! As well as not standing in blue light – the apps are free! The most valuable nuts are some of the cheapest! Pumpkin seeds – 80% protein! To make live food – seeds for sprouts cost 80 cents. Or 1.99 leva to buy thyme in a pot and put it in your salad!

"Training is a pleasure for which I do not have the time and finances!" On YouTube – there are thousands of free videos. Our site has a campaign – "Stand Yourself Up in 6 Weeks"! You didn't ask! Because it's easier! The best dancers in the world have learned from the internet!

On March 25, 2018, I was at a lecture on food supplements, which was supposed to be informative! The woman there said that the supplement saves us the need to breathe! You will give 77 leva every 20 days for a jar of seaweed, but you will not learn to breathe?!

A month ago, I talked to another food supplement company. The lady I talked to said the same thing – people do not have time to think about what they eat and how they move. The powder in the jar is easier! One spoon and there you go! I have not heard about someone on supplements being of low metabolic age! And I found representatives of all sorts of supplements and guess what – no one is at a minimum!

People are living in such a way that they will pass on before getting their last salary! And as if they don't mind! At the age of 30 we have already forgotten to live. At 45 we pass away from stress, heart attack or diabetes. And in the best case we start taking blood pressure pills from 40 years of age. Why???

It is not normal!!! Look around! Look around and see how everyone is like that! It is not normal! Two generations ago, people lived for 99–110 years. Now the average life expectancy is 66 years for women. Enough. And when I listen to the grandmothers in our neighborhood, the pension is barely enough for medicine. How could you not want to die before that!

Every day I see new faces in the gym. And every day I see statistics: 30 years old, and with a metabolic age of 58 years! If the average duration is 66 years, you are 58 years old in tissues and organs. Congratulations – you have 8 more years! How do you like it?!?

For 10 years I have been repeating how the skin is a mirror of what is inside us! And for 8 months I noticed that it is already written in magazines, on the Internet, in articles and everywhere! I admit – I'm really happy! And I believe that after another 20–30 everyone will understand it! And I know I will be alive to see this. And not just alive, but with tight skin without a wrinkle, pumped ass, flat stomach and legs without cellulite! And most importantly – I will be 60 years old, and inside I will be 19.

Everyone chooses who to follow! Who to look like! Try to be yourself! Prove to yourself that you are the best version!

You choose whether to be healthy or to be among the sheep!

P.S. The experience is to share! That's why I share it with you. I hope you will read something that will make you think.

Wonderful day, Lovely one! In 30 years, if you have nothing to do, call me so we can go jogging on the beach.

Beauty is an inner feeling that reflects in the mirror.

Emiliya Belcheva

YO-YO: I Lose Weight, I Gain Weight ... Again and Again

Eighty percent of success is just showing up.

Woody Allen

Sounds familiar?

Have you noticed that you gain weight in specific months! No matter what you eat! For example, I started gaining from the sixth month of my first pregnancy and every year in January, I gain weight! Then I got pregnant a second time. Now I gain weight at the end of November and the end of January. It took me 3 years to stop the cycle!

The body is like a book. If something happens, it remembers it. To prevent panic at the last minute, set it as your phone's alarm and remind yourself. Many women experience contractions on the day of birth years after giving birth. I am a living example! Depression around the time of the period... the desire to eat sweets... it's coded. You get sad and boom! Ingenious insight – eat sweets!

We make the habit easy! It's hard to break it! Find out when it happens and start working on it, but 2–3 weeks in advance!

A few examples:

The body does not react immediately! It needs time. Let's see the cycle. The same thing is repeated every month. Just... we need more calories and eating 5–7 days before the start of our period. If we need 1,300 calories normally, these days the calories are 1,500. The period in which we are irritated, sad and loving. This is usually the period when we are not to be talked to. But by the time the body understands it, our period has already begun. When it comes to us, we need fewer calories! But the brain thinks we should eat. It sends a signal and we start robbing the refrigerator. At this point we need 1,100–1,200 calories. We are already unloading! And what do we do? We eat 3 chocolate bars, French fries, ice cream, waffles... about 2,500 calories! So what? Only double. And then we feel surprised we gain weight and bloat. For as long as I know this, I never bloat during my period! I don't swell! I'm not grumpy! Nobody understands that I'm on my period! And I'm as productive as on other days.

My advice on this is: 4–5 days before the period, eat a little bit more fat than usual.

The same is in the period winter through to summer. Winter begins. We eat dead food. A lot of positive charge. We are getting older. We eat volume, not quality. We stretch the stomach. We get used to eating huge portions. Spring is coming. If in the winter we needed 200–300 calories on top to keep warm, another 100 to compensate for the lack of vitamin D, etc., then in the spring we want to unload. Instead of 1,600 calories, we need 1,100 calories. Many people do not gain weight in winter but namely in the months of February–March–April! Hello, summer! Hello, big ass! The body has entered a cycle and will not come out for a month. Your belly will not shrink in 2 weeks. As the weather changes, so does your diet. By changing your lifestyle and stress, you will also need a change in your diet. Don't wait to gain weight to realize it.

The same mistake is made with activities. You haven't exercised until now; you've used 1,200 calories. The next moment you start training. You liquefy fat and use it (extra calories). You increase your appetite from training. Your brain tells you, "You're training – eat more." From everything you do, your calorie intake rises by 200 to 300 calories. Your body is hungry for fat and protein. And you give it fast carbs and sugars. You need cement and I give you carboard! What happens then? Your need becomes about 1,500 calories a day. And you eat 2,800. You actually start eating more calories than when you didn't exercise! How do you want to lose weight? And most importantly: how do you want not to gain weight?

The body remembers! You should remember this too! And every hesitation in your weight is remembered! So don't say: "So what, just 2–3 kilos more." Every year you will gain 2–3 and you will not lose them! Until they become 20–30 when what you will do is give up! You have no idea how many such cases I work with.

Think about what you eat! Eat more live food than dead!!!

Regenerate, do not kill yourself!

Feel your body! And don't ignore it! This is your temple! This is your place! And only you can take care of it!

A magical day, Wonderful!

Take care of your body. It's the only place you have to live.

Jim Rohn

Collagen Plus Homemade Collagen Recipe

I was very happy when yesterday Didi told me: "The article got very popular, you need to write a collagen recipe!"

So, let's begin.

Do you know what collagen is? Imagine a very beautiful girl. She has long brown hair. Today she braided it. You see perfectly how the three strands intertwine. Sunlight is reflected in the brown color. It is so shiny and alive that you want to touch it and pull it to see how healthy it is. It is elastic to the touch and the moment you release it from your hand, it stands again in a perfectly arranged chain, without a single protruding hair.

Well, that's what collagen looks like. It is composed of three protein chains forming a braid. When the three are together, it is hard and strong as steel. Thirty-three percent of the proteins in our body are collagen. Bone, muscles, tendons and 75% of the skin are made of collagen.

To see the whole picture and connections, let's look in depth.

There are cells in the skin called fibroblasts (it always sounds like something from Star Wars). These are special skin cells located in the dermis. They in turn produce elastin (which gives elasticity) and glucosaminoglycan (which gives hydration). In addition, they also produce procollagen (short-chain collagen). From them, grouping together, they form complete collagen molecules again. But secondary factors also intervene here. Hyaluronic acid is needed to bind elastin to collagen. Thus, vitamin C is involved in many of the stages. In the absence of vitamin C, collagen synthesis is disrupted.

For bones, everyone says, "drink calcium"! Yes, but no! The main protein in bones is collagen. It binds to calcium and phosphorus, and forms a strong structure. Imagine it as glue. If you have papers of different colors but you don't have glue.... you can't create anything!!! In the absence of "glue" we have –

sagging skin, wrinkles, hair loss, cellulite, digestive problems, joint pain and many other consequences.

Why cellulite and stretch marks? When we have collagen in the skin, it is elastic. Something like a brand-new legging. It tightens, lifts the ass, everything looks perfect! Yes, just like the black one in the closet! But, if the legging starts to wear off from wearing it, when we put it on, the situation is different, isn't it? All the defects are visible, it no longer tightens, but sags.

Collagen in the joints is something like the icing on a cake. It allows us to keep everything in place and move like "honey and butter."

What do the amino acids contained in collagen actually do?

Glycine – does not allow thinning of muscles and cartilage, stimulates regeneration, supports liver function.

Lysine – is involved in bone formation. It is also responsible for the absorption of calcium and nitrogen and ensures that this process proceeds normally.

Proline – guarantees the strength of collagen fibers, which are related to the normal condition of the heart, skin and all cartilage. Decomposes fat deposits in the circulatory system.

Glutamic acid – acts as a neurotransmitter. How does it affect the intestines?

Taking collagen with food is like taking your car to have a flat tire fixed. It fills the injured area (inflammation). And it's like glue poured on top. Makes the intestines thicker and healthier. The amino acids in collagen make up the tissue that lines the colon and gastrointestinal tract. So, they help with acid reflux, Crohn's disease, colitis, lazy bowels and many other problems.

If you have split nails – this is also a lack of collagen. It is involved in the construction of nails, hair and teeth.

Collagen increases metabolism and muscle mass. This is due to the smallest amino acid in our body, contained in collagen. Glycine is responsible for building muscle mass. And everyone knows that after a certain age it is very difficult! We are not talking about fat, but about muscle! It plays an important role in the digestive and central nervous systems.

Glycine also helps protect the liver. We depend on it to improve blood flow and its quality. In the consumption of all "harmful substances" it is glycine that helps keep your heart young and prevent liver problems.

Another important amino acid in collagen is proline. It is responsible for breaking down fat deposits in the bloodstream and reducing their buildup.

There is controversy over how many types of collagens are in the human body. Some claim that there are 16, others 25. In reality, there are 6 main types: type 1,2,3,4,5 and 10.

"The body can do anything. It is the mind we need to convince."

Type 1 – 90% of collagen in the human body. It builds tendons, ligaments, organs, skin, bones and is located in the gastrointestinal tract. It holds the fabric together and does not allow it to break.

Type 2 – forms cartilage.

Type 3 – these are reticular fibers. Or simply put – a network. Remember Grandma's shopping bag from 20–30 years ago? It's all mesh, and some models only had rubber on the handles? This type is involved in the organs, skin, blood vessels and heart. It is usually found in combination with Type 1.

With type 3 breakdown and lack of collagen, we have weak blood vessels, varicose veins and a risk of premature death (heart attack, stroke and the like).

Type 4 – something like stretch film. It is found in endothelial cells. They form tissues that surround organs, muscles and fat (something like stretch film). The main plates are in the nerves and blood vessels. They participate in our digestive organs and respiratory surfaces. Between the skin and the underlying tissue (fat or muscle). As here it is similar to a fluid (thick liquid).

Type 5 – builds the surface of cells, hair, placenta.

Type 10 – helps to form bones and articular cartilage. Updated every year.

I don't expect you to remember 50% of the information you read. My goal was to make you realize how important collagen is for your body! And having wrinkles, cellulite or cracked skin is your least problem. If by the age of 40 only half of humanity has complaints, by the age of 50 the sufferers are already 75%, and by the age of 70 – 90%. It all starts with your food!

What destroys collagen?

1. Age – at the age of 30 the real aging of the bones begins. The processes of breakdown of collagen fibers prevail over the processes of synthesis. Menopause in women is another criterion. It reduces the absorption of trace elements and vitamins that stimulate collagen synthesis. We start eating saltier (remember the salt texts, right?).

2. Free radicals, toxins and the enzyme collagenase systematically attack and destroy collagen fibers. We have already commented on it separately.

3. Heredity – weak collagen predisposes to inflammatory processes, tumors, osteoporosis. This is already being analyzed with iris diagnostics. The iris is made up of connective tissue. If there are many dips and dents, it is considered low quality collagen fibers.

4. Ultraviolet rays – they cause the breakdown of collagen fibers and artificial aging. To prevent this from happening, UVA and UVB rays should be avoided.

5. Sugar – increases the rate of glycation – a process in which blood sugars attach to proteins to form new molecules (AGEs). They damage nearby proteins and make collagen dry, brittle and weak.

6. Food – the wrong food causes an avalanche of collagen chains. Just like sugar.
7. Smoking – the chemicals present in cigarettes cause the breakdown of elastin and collagen in the skin. Nicotine narrows blood vessels. Reduces blood and nutrient flow. Muscles eat themselves to survive.

Women between the ages of 35 and 55 need about 5–7 grams of collagen a day, and actively training individuals need 10 grams of collagen hydrolysate.

Collagen sources

1. Collagen from beef, turkey – they have high concentration of stable collagen fibers. Mostly collagen is Type 1 and Type 3. Rich in glycine and proline. Supports creatine production. Stimulates the production of its own collagen. Sheep and pork are also Type 1, but with lower stability of collagen fibers.
2. Chicken and rabbit collagen – the richest in Type 2. Most suitable for building cartilage. Most supplements use chicken collagen. Unfortunately, during the heat treatment of meat, most of the collagen fibers break down.
3. Fish collagen – mainly Type 1. Easily absorbed by the body. Contains glycine. Proline and hydroxyproline. With low hydroxyproline there is a degradation of the joints. Must be taken with vitamin C!
4. Collagen in eggshells – also contains mainly collagen Type 1. But it also contains types 3, 4 and 10. Approximately 100 more of type 1 than types 3, 4 or 10.
5. The richest in collagen among plants is wheat. We are not talking about bread!

How to absorb collagen and slow down the breakdown processes

We should take vitamin C regularly. Fruit or fruit juice with a high content of vitamin C guarantees the absorption of collagen! The daily dose is 75 mg of vitamin C. Studies have shown that this vitamin can increase collagen synthesis up to 8 times. Regular intake of vitamins C, A, D, E are important for its processing. This can also be as an intake of antioxidants (vitamin A, vitamin C and vitamin E). They neutralize free radicals and help eliminate them from the body.

Eat nuts. They have no collagen! But they have a lot of vitamins and minerals that you need.

Another way to increase collagen synthesis is regular exfoliation with fruit acids (alpha and polyhydroxy). They break down the connections between the cells of the stratum corneum (the top layer of the skin) and help remove dead cells. Contained in each fruit.

Another way is with the help of peptides. Some products for external use contain them. Something like an external irritant that causes the skin to synthesize collagen.

I am often asked, "Should I drink gelatin?" Collagen is different from gelatin. Gelatin is obtained from collagen after its breakdown. This is how bone broth works. After a long cooking, collagen breaks down. It goes into the water and we drink it. This decay is from 24 to 48 hours. Gelatin in stores is obtained from various additives, you really do not know what it is! And what is homemade is always better!

Beauty starts from within. If you have beautiful skin, then you have collagen, elastin, hyaluronic acid, vitamins and minerals. And that means you're as strong inside as a concrete block! To make collagen, you need vitamin C, lysine and proline. Egg whites and wheat sprouts are rich in proline. Meat, fish, nuts – lysine. Algae and magnesium-rich foods stimulate the synthesis of hyaluronic acid. And then they bind to elastin, and so on.

And as I promised a "homemade collagen recipe":

Fill the pot with bones to the top. If they do not have meat, the broth will be rich in more minerals. If there is meat, there will be more amino acids. Fill a few fingers under the rim of the pot with water. At 12 liters put 1 cup of apple cider vinegar and let sit for 1 hour (if you have indigestion and vinegar does not affect you well, skip it). You can add onions, garlic, celery, parsley. Some protein and mixed metabolic types may be sensitive to the number of vegetables added. Therefore, for the first time I recommend not to use them. Let it simmer on a low heat. It should not boil! Boiling destroys many important ingredients. The longer we simmer, the more nutrients will come out of the bones in the broth. Fish bones need 4 to 24 hours. Chicken – from 6 to 34 hours. Pork – from 12 to 48 hours. Veal – from 12 to 72 hours. After cooking it, leave it on the hot plate. When it cools, remove the bones and pieces, pour into jars (made of glass!), But not to the top. Cool and freeze. Drink 1 tsp. per day. And maybe more. It is an ideal base for soups. The more gelled the broth, the better.

It is good to do a course of 6–8 weeks, twice a year with one glass a day. But it's not bad to drink when we want. Do not wait for a deficit. Prevent the problem, don't wait for it to appear to cure it!

Smile! Because you attract what you are.

How Many Times a Week Should I Exercise for Good Results?

There are 24 hours in a day, in a week – 168 hours. According to a survey conducted in 2016, each person spends an average of 11 years of his life on the Internet! Everyone spends at least an hour in pointless scrolling a day on a social network! A woman spends over 40 minutes to an hour every day over the sink and dishes, not to mention cleaning, cooking and everything else. How much time a day do we waste on smoking cigarettes or pointless things? If in 168 hours we can't find 4 hours for us, why do we live?

How often do you eat? If you eat properly, then every 4 to 6 hours. Do not starve for 3 days and then overeat until bursting! In the same way, you can't set aside 2 hours for training from 168 hours and expect a result.

Why do we exercise?

To change the way your body works! The meaning of a workout is not to kill ourselves in an hour and resuscitate for 4 days! The meaning of a workout is to teach us how to move properly in our daily lives! The workout is one small dot in the big circle. After that, you should feel the change in your body, not stiffness. If you have a stoop, then be straighter with ease. During the training itself, you can feel where there is a twist and where the problem is.

When the trainer says, "You have to feel something somewhere" this is not to be missed! He says it to make sure you give him feedback. If you feel it, you are training properly!

If not, in the best case you will train for 2 years and you will not have improvement. In the worst case... you will hunch even more and get injured. There is a difference between "hear" and "listen."

Every time someone comes to a workout for the first time I tell them:

1–2 times a week is for mental relief,

2–3 is for tone and cheerful mood and

4 times is the minimum to lose weight and adjust posture and habits.

His eyes become "pancake-like" as if I'm saying he needs to get to the moon. More than 1,000,000 excuses come immediately – and the answer is, "I can't." I always ask – you don't have time or? And they start – I can't leave the child with anybody (we have a free children's corner), yes, but I do not know how I will manage to come from work etc.

We can always find an excuse! If we find an excuse, the result is not what we want.

So, before you start, ask yourself, "What do I want?" And then answer the even more important question, "Why do I want it?" Because I want it to be easier for me so I don't have pain or because others think I'm fat...

Don't do something you don't want to do!

And do not look for excuses!

Even since I have been saying "no" more, my life has become better.

Life is an endless workout! Use it!

Some people say they don't have time to go to the gym. What a distortion.

Stephen Covey

Trick or Treat? Alkalinity versus Acidity

Great people have will, weak ones have wishes.

Chinese proverb

I don't like age, but I like evidence in numbers. It is amazing how the cause of cancer was discovered in 1921. In 1931, the German scientist Otto Heinrich Warburg received the Nobel Prize for his work! He proves that through our diet and exercise we change our body from an alkaline to acidic environment. As lack of oxygen in the cells causes an acidic environment, decreasing oxygen and increasing acidity in the body go hand in hand. A really acidic environment is an oxygen-free environment.

Healthy cells without 35% oxygen can be transformed into a cancer cell in just two days!

All cells need oxygen to live. Only cancer cells can live without oxygen. Really, what's going on? We deprive the body of oxygen (distorted posture, shallow breathing). We do even more damage with bad food (white flour, sugar, white salt, dairy products, juices, chips and what not) to become an acidic environment. And the body has no choice but to mutate.

Cancer is the result of the body's adaptation to our way of life! Not a disease!

Remember the article on free radicals? When we are alkaline, our body's charge is negative. When we are acidic, the charge is positive. Plants have a minus 450 charge. We humans have a minus 70 charge. Nature invented it – you eat fresh food and recharge! You eat dead food (including a lot of cooked food) and you take your charge away. Everything after being picked from its roots begins to decompose. From negative -450, the charge becomes positive to +650. You choose whether to fill your stomach and grow old or to have eternal youth.

Youth is beauty! Youth is health in tissues and organs. What is time? Something with which we have measured the way our lives go. Why are there animals and trees that live longer than others? The place is the same for everyone! Their way of life is different!

Let's get back to food. Depending on proteins, carbohydrates, fats, vitamins and minerals, conditions of acidity or alkalinity are created in the body. In other words, it all depends on what you eat. The acidic or alkaline state is measured with a pH whose values range from 0 to 14, where 7 is the neutral zone. From 0 to 7 is an acidic environment, and from 7 to 14 is alkaline.

How do acidic or alkaline foods affect health? In order to function successfully, the cells should be in the pH range just above 7. A healthy person has a pH in the blood between 7.4 and 7.45. If someone's pH is below 7, that person falls into a coma. Cancer cells begin to develop in the human body when the pH drops below 6.2. Remember the article about water and eternal youth? PH was one of the factors we had to monitor. Why? Because it exhausted us and disturbed the environment, if it is above or below what is necessary!

You get in now, right?

Motivation gets you started. Habit is what makes you go on.

Jim Ryan

The food that makes you acidic is: refined sugar and all its derivatives, all dairy, refined salt (including Himalayan), refined flour and all its derivatives (pasta, cakes, biscuits), roasted nuts, margarine, caffeine (coffee, black tea, chocolate), alcohol, cigarettes, any cooked food (heat treatment destroys oxygen and increases the acidity of food), cans that contain preservatives, artificial colors, flavors, stabilizers and much more. Only coarse sea salt (it is gray and looks fatty in the package, it is not fine) is useful for you.

The important thing here is "Which food helps you alkalize?"

All fresh fruits and vegetables. Raw vegetables produce oxygen, unlike heat-treated ones. And fruits produce a lot of oxygen.

Water is important for oxygen production. Chronic stress is very important and is the cause of most degenerative diseases.

Upright posture – allows the flow of oxygen throughout the body. Habits are the way to control our body!

Movement gives oxygen to the whole body. A sedentary lifestyle is ruining your health! And don't make excuses here – I don't have time! I have two children aged 2 and 3, my husband is running errands all day and I manage to be a housewife, to work (to lead personal consultations, trainings, to write not one, but two books, to maintain a blog, to answer your questions and what not?). And I still find time for myself! How? I made it a habit. An hour a day is for me! It's all up to you! It's not your husband, it's not your work, it's not the children! It is your personal choice. Remember the last nonsense you bought and you still feel bad about – a bag, clothes, shoes, cosmetics. Something that you really regret buying. You had no money for it and yet somehow you found the money and bought it. How? By depriving yourself of something else. This is your choice. Isn't health your priority? When was the last time you thought about yourself and not everybody around you? I think you get me. One of my rules in life is: take care of yourself first and then others. If I don't feel okay, I can't take care of my children when they need me; I will burden them. This is why it is better to have a sink full of dishes, lots of laundry, dirty floors for a day instead of neglecting myself!

To be healthy, we must mostly eat alkaline food! Or compensate with proper breathing! Always, if one is lame, another compensates. The problem is that today many things are lame and there is nothing to compensate with!!!

Today, there are three ways to treat cancer – surgery, radiation therapy and chemotherapy. None of the methods guarantees a cure. At the same time, every method causes side effects. But not like those in the pill leaflets; Serious side effects! Doctors say it is in remission. Why? Because they cut the dead tissue, the mutated tissue. But the button is already pressed. We do not stand up. We are not starting to move. We are hunching even more. We are careful not to move, not to breathe, not to do something. And suddenly – there are dissipations throughout the body! How did it happen?

Treatment of cancer by changing the pH is not invasive. You remember all those articles – "Miracle, he went to the Himalayas and defeated cancer!" The lesson of this story is that one should check the pH of his body. If you are diagnosed with cancer, it is very likely that your pH is below 6.2. If the pH is less than 6.5 it is already dangerous to health It is a slightly acidic pH and the level of oxygen in the blood is reduced, increased carbon dioxide levels. Lack of oxygen in the blood increases free radicals. Free radicals, improper food, overexcitement, poor focus, etc. We are aging artificially. At the age of 20 we have the organs of 90-year-olds!

Everyone says, "I don't have time!" You choose whether you will spend some time now and live until 120 or you will be almost dead at 60. How often do you go to your grandparents? What about your parents? Why? Because you have nothing to do with them! Why? Because they are old! Why? Because of their way of life! My mother is over 50 and do you know what I do with her? Everything! She comes to trainings with me! We go to discos! We go out shopping. She spends all night driving because she was at a party somewhere in the country. She wasn't always like that! She had no energy before. She had no strength. And someone will say, "She's a free woman!" Not really! She is at work all day. From 09:00 to 20:00. She carries thousands of things on her shoulders. She works 24/7.

The difference is that she started moving, eating right and everything changed!

It is up to you! Everything is in your hands! There are people who just gave up – it's the story of my life, I don't have time, my time has passed... It is all in your head. In my head thoughts are like this – life is ahead of me, I achieved so much by the time I am 30, I have another 90 years up front.

In fact, with the time spent on health (for sports, for preparing food for work) you gain time in the future! Health is not bought when you need it. It is taken in advance! Something like a loan. This does not happen with a list at the end of the article. This comes with a long explanation of what, how and why. That's why I write an article every day for "good morning." I splash you with cold water, slap you and hope you wake up. Separate yourself from the crowd and don't walk among the sheep. Why sheep? Because they follow the others. And the others are on their way to the abyss.

And you? How are you today?

The Deception

You can't win or lose if you don't participate.

David Bowie

Yesterday at my personal consultation with Egi we talked about collagen. And I remembered how many things we do in halves. Not because we don't want to, but because we don't know. We take supplements that have been recommended to us, and we do not know that we do not absorb them due to another lack. So, in the first place we burden our body, in the second – we throw money to the wind. Last but not least, we make efforts and time that no one seems to appreciate. Result = zero. Then why do we want to do it again?

When we make an effort and do not see a result, we have no incentive to do it again! Right?

When we take collagen in any form, we definitely need vitamin C! If we take iron, we also can't absorb it without vitamin C.

Let's see what vitamin C actually does and what mistakes we should not make?

I'll start with part of the lesson: Vitamin C (ascorbic acid) is not synthesized in the body. We have to get it on the side. If we get it with a pill, the quality is often unsatisfactory. The body replenishes the necessary stock with low quality and if we eat a lemon after that (high quality), it does not process it. It says, "I've had enough, throw the newcomer in the trash." And we pee on it. That's why it's good if you take vitamin C in the evening. This will not affect what we eat during the day. It will only add to it.

Vitamin C has a strong antioxidant effect which means that it fights free radicals in the body – the causes of cancer and many other diseases. Vitamin C cleans slag and toxins. If combined with vitamins E and A it becomes a health bomb. Something like a waterfall. It catches you and cleanses you from scratch. Vitamins A, E and C are interrelated. Each increases the strength of the other. Something like Batman, Batgirl and Robin. In itself, each one is good. But together... hmm...

When I worked as a beautician, I always mixed vitamin C, Retinoid (vitamin A), vitamin E and collagen. The faces of my clients were rejuvenated by 10–20 years with one procedure. The problem was that they did not eat properly and did not get vitamins from the inside. So, the skin was saturated, literally soaked, but for a month. Their food was breaking down collagen bonds. And the next month again and again, and again, and again... Sounds familiar?

Did you understand the collagen pages well? Vitamin C stimulates collagen synthesis. Exactly 33% of the proteins in your body are collagen. You have it in muscles, bones, skin, organs... it is everywhere! No vitamin C, no collagen. You're getting old! Your quality is falling! The quality of your tissues and organs. Your quality of sleep. Your quality of functioning. Your quality of life! You don't want it, do you?

You have collagen – you have no wounds. Vitamin C helps heal wounds. A wound does not necessarily mean torn skin. It may be a scar, it may be stretch marks, it may be stretched skin from rapid weight gain or loss.

One in three suffers from iron deficiency. We drink pills, supplements, ampoules, take injections, eat nettles, and do we combine it with vitamin C? No vitamin C – no absorption of iron. Iron is in the tissues, teeth, bones.

Which foods are richest in vitamin C? Not lemons! Rosehips have 1,250 mg per 100 g, and citrus fruits only 50 mg per 100 g. I love baobab fruits. They are sold crushed and put in a smoothie or taken with tea. Their powder has a slightly sour taste and is very fresh. There are 350 mg in 100 g, in a daily dose of 15 g there are 52 mg. I also like rosehip flour, but since I don't cook anything with dough, I stopped using it for pastries. Now I add it to the morning smoothie for breakfast.

However, there is a trick! Vitamin C dies from heat treatment and speed! Many people make fresh carrots and citrus because of vitamin C. When the juicer is turned quickly, vitamin C is oxidized by the air. This oxidation turns it into dehydroascorbate. It oxidizes in the same way when left for 2–3 hours in a cup or the tablet has been opened to moisture and oxygen. If vitamin C keeps the cells young, alive and healthy, dehydroascorbate damages them!

Heat treatment destroys it, as well as many other useful elements in our food. Therefore, I recommend it to be eaten raw!

Another big plus is its assistance in the transfer of oxygen to the brain. That's how the brain is alive!

When we catch a cold, the first thing we drink is vitamin C! Why? Because in addition to being an antioxidant, it increases the strength and number of white blood cells in the blood. They have the function of detecting, destroying and eating viruses, bacteria and cancer cells.

The color of your skin depends on vitamin C! Want white radiant skin without imperfections? It needs oxygen, exercise and vitamin C! You want to shrink pores, burn acne and remove fine wrinkles – smear the face every day with lemon, stay like this for 20 minutes and rinse.

The purpose of each of my articles or chapters in the book is not to memorize all things after reading, but to acquire a habit which you don't think about all the time. When eating something to get iron, calcium or collagen, always take vitamin C. If you eat spinach, dock, bone broth or dairy, add something sour (citrus, rosehips or other). If you eat meat and you feel heavy, add lemon. The acid will break down the food quickly, you will absorb what you need and you're done. But if it's something light and you add lemon... you'll get hungry fast!

Smiling and a fresh day, Irresistible!

My advice to you is not to inquire why or whither, but just enjoy your ice cream while it's on your plate.

Thornton Wilder

How to Be 100% Motivated
24 Hours/365 Days!

Have you noticed how children celebrate each victory? And they are happy to the fullest that they jumped over the puddle, that they turned on the tap themselves, that they managed to brush their teeth and all sorts of little things that were insignificant to us.

That's where the key to success is!

To understand why, we need to get to know the hormone dopamine!

Often called the hormone of motivation.

Dopamine is a hormone that is formed in our body. It has peaks and drops or so-called dopamine activity. It is the key to the mental processes of motivation and concentration. Addiction to psychotropic substances, from nicotine and alcohol to heroin, as well as gambling addiction, come from this direction. What does cocaine do? Stimulates the synthesis of dopamine or in other words increased dopamine activity – over-motivation.

When dopamine activity decreases, there comes a moment of unpreparedness, depression, insecurity, procrastination. Permanent deficiency develops Parkinson's disease and many other motor deficits and diseases. And with a constant increase – schizophrenia. This is not a ping pong ball, don't play with it. Either keep it up or keep it down.

The choice is yours!

Detoxification – occurs in the presence of dopamine. In addition to motivation, it is responsible for the amount of blood entering and filtering in the kidneys, respectively, and pumped by the heart. With an increased amount of dopamine, the blood vessels open, with a reduced amount they close.

Dopamine is an intermediate from which adrenaline is produced.

So, celebrate every victory, no matter how small it is!

It doesn't have to be a spectacular celebration of success. Every experienced satisfaction, satisfaction or even a slight applause of yourself makes you release dopamine. Increase your motivation at every opportunity! It is no coincidence that at the end of each workout we clap! We don't applaud me! Everybody applauds themselves. The more satisfied you are with what you give during training, the more you clap.

Every day be better than the day before!

The skill is what you are capable of. Motivation determines what you do. Attitude determines how well you do it.

Louis Holtz

What Should I Eat?

In recent weeks, this has been the main question asked of me!
I can't tell you what to eat! I can tell you what not to eat!
White flour, sugar, salt (only gray sea greasy salt is good), dairy
products! And you come to ask me: "Still, what should I eat?"
Everything!
Years ago, I was fighting bacteria and I was forbidden
to eat the above "foods." During the first month it was
too difficult. I read the labels and realized that they are in
everything I was used to. Hell no!!! I was reading recipes in
forums etc. I was amazed how everything healthy is made
with super expensive products! On top of that, the drugs were
super expensive and were taken for a long time! Every time I
ate something harmful, I felt sick. At one point I thought it's
my guilty conscience. Until my brother opened my eyes and
explained to me that I feed this bacterium with the products
described above. That's how it becomes strong. And when I
take an antibiotic, it releases substances that make me sick.
Actually, it was the bacteria that was poisoning me. Only
because I wanted to survive is why I gathered my will not to
eat! Why should I poison my body and waste my money when
I can just stop eating rubbish!?
Then I realized I didn't need expensive recipes! People
who constantly upload recipes about how they made another
healthy dessert do not eat properly! If you give value to your
body, you don't eat sweet! You don't think about desserts!
You don't think about how to make a cake or pastry just to
eat something that your brain doesn't judge you for. You don't
even think of sweet!

If you want to extend your life, reduce the food.
Benjamin Franklin

129

How to eat? Depending on your metabolic type – between 4 and 6 hours. But if you eat more often than every 4 hours – you do not give value! Value for me is one thing, for you it is another, for Mimka, it is a third. If you lack minerals (you constantly eat something salty), then minerals are of value to you. If you want sour (you lack enzymes), then enzymes are a value for you. If you want to eat too much sweets, one of the reasons is lack of fat in your diet. Fat equals energy etc.

The idea is this: if you have 4 hours from breakfast to noon, you don't have to think about food at that time – candy, coffee, nothing! Only water! The idea is to eat so that you do not deprive yourself. Not to starve in order to spend 4 hours without food.

Valuable food satisfies you for 4 hours. If you are a carbohydrate type, it can be in 6 hours. Food is the greatest pleasure, do not deprive yourself of it!

Food determines what we are!

Today Geri and I talked about water. If we do not drink water, the first dehydration occurs in our brain! The spine is distorted. We become unproductive! For a job that we can do in 30 minutes, we need 4 hours. There is no concentration. As if we are not here! She said, "I don't like water." What's going on? Water doesn't have the minerals she needs. The body processes a consumable that exhausts it, not gives it value. The body is not stupid! It stops wanting that consumable.

Instead, we need to add a little salt. You already know which one! Not Himalayan, not white, not in salt shaker! The water is saturated with minerals and you're fine! Before your period, do you get nervous? Well, you lack fat – you lack good cholesterol.

Everything in the conversations starts with this, "How to lower your metabolic age?" It is very complex! It depends on what you eat, what kind of water you drink, when do you go to bed, how much you sleep, how do you stand, how do you breathe... everything! Don't bother changing everything! Because in two weeks you will give up! I love numbers. In 10 years (12 months x 24 working days x 10 people a day x 10 years) about 28,800 people have passed through my hands. Furthermore, I have 20–30-people classes, I lecture 60–100 people and about 25 people pass a day through my parlor in high season. At some Masterclasses I lecture 450–500 people. I know when a person acts and when they give up! Don't give up! Be active!

It is very easy!

Just try it!

Try to monitor how you feel after each meal. You don't need a psychologist to understand how you feel!

Be happy! Be yourself!

Many people skip happiness not because they didn't find it, but because they didn't slow down to enjoy it.

William Feather

How Often Do You Poop?

Many people blush here! But admit it! You pray to God to go poop so you can feel better! The intestines of women, the uterus, the ovaries, if we have given birth and rearranged ourselves... it is a horror! 1–2 times a week is a holiday! Am I right?

I was like that myself. And I'm not afraid to say it! After the births it was horror, Pain, toxins! It was like I was poisoned! I was poisoned in fact! Ever since I straightened my posture and changed my diet, I have been reborn!

The truth is that we have to go to the small happy room as many times as we eat minus 1. If you eat 4 times, then 3 times you need to poop. Otherwise, you keep the food longer than necessary and get toxic.

Think what a dead animal smells like in a few days! What if you keep food in the warm? Lentils get spoiled in 5–6 hours. Yes... you get me, right? Say yes! I know it is like this! I will ask you as you read, that if you agree with something I said, to say yes. When you agree, your brain accepts it and puts it into routine tasks! But more on that in another page.

Why is it important to clean up? You already know that the distance from the mouth to the anus is from 7 to 14 meters. It depends on your ancestors, not you. Where they lived and accordingly determines your metabolic type. And for the ignorant – this is whether digestible protein comes from meat or from plants. To make it clear to you, I will give you the following example. We will set time for easier calculations. If the length is the hours, then the meat is digested in 7 hours. If it's in you after the seventh, it gets toxic. The plant is absorbed between the seventh and fourteenth. So, if you are a protein type and you eat a lot of carbohydrates, you are a "real gut." Think of such acquaintances. They eat but they don't get fat. They do not digest! They throw it away before the protein molecule is extracted!

You don't have to hold back. Food after certain hours poisons you! It's like eating something spoiled! That's why you feel irritated, sick, heavy, etc.

The idea is as follows:

If you are hunched over, you crush your intestines. Imagine filling a sausage. If someone squeezes the intestine (or now it's called an organic bag), the minced meat cannot pass. It begins to stretch and if it is inside you, it hurts. If it stretches, then instead of collecting 500 grams, it will collect a kilogram. And you don't push it out. You're holding back again!

If you have a stomach, more precisely you do not have a tight lower abdominal wall, then you have nothing to push. It is repeated again. Like a stretched sock that can fit both feet. And what happens – you wait until everything overflows. The glass is empty after it is full! Intestines become lazy and clogged!

All my life I have trained for the upper abdominal six pack. Yes, I have a six pack! To be one of the strong and cool ones! I did 100 pushups every day, another 100 side pushups, then I grabbed a machine or levers and lifted my legs up... so far everything was for the upper abdominal wall. On top of that, I did them wrong... but that's another topic!

The lower abdominal wall is from your groin to your navel! This is where you want to be muscly! If you are not flat there (bones are the lateral bones protruding at the upper end of the triangle), then you retain feces.

If you don't have fiber – and not the ones in the packets, then you have nothing to help digest the food. Do you remember the chickens? They eat pebbles, entering the mill helps them grind. Your stones are the fibers. There is fiber in living food – fruits and vegetables. Fiber is what's left after you squeeze fresh juice. Your body does the same. You eat an apple; it is digested in the stomach and goes to the intestines. The intestines are like the tentacles of an octopus, like a suction cup. It sucks in the necessary squeezed juice, and the rest is pushed into the intestines and comes out. If there is no fiber, there is nothing to help get rid of unnecessary substances.

Did you understand? Yes, right?

I love examples, I remember more easily with them!

To help ourselves, we need to make a few things a habit

* Eat more live food (fiber) than dead! And if you buy a packet of fibers, do not rely only on it! It will help you for a month, then it will not work again.
* Think about how you sit. Do not cross your legs! Do not sit with your stomach pushed inwards!
* Work on the lower abdominal wall. Once again, I remind you that our site has a free campaign "Stand Yourself Up in 6 Weeks" – the second week we show you an exercise for it!
* Drink water! 0.033 liters per kilogram.
* Don't hold it in! Teach your gut that you will respond! Otherwise, it will not work when you want it to.

It is right to get up in the morning, empty and then eat again. After breakfast, go again. The trapped food pushes out the residue and you cleanse. So, you're productive all day! In the afternoon, around 4–5 p.m. you should go again. Just like babies do – they eat, they poop and again and again…

Bottled Juices and More

They keep asking me, "But what do you have against bottled juice?" I have something against some! Let's see.

The fruits are picked and then bought by another company. Its purpose is to extract the juice from the fruit. The problem is that if you just press it on a horizontal press, you will get only 60% of the juice contained. Everyone is pursuing their own interest! To increase the volume of the final product, the fruit is squeezed by hot pressing with screw presses. You know, when we boil the fruit, it softens which equals more juice. But here we raise the yield to 70%.

In order to reach 85–90% yield of the final product, it is further processed before pressing with enzymes. Bulgarian chemicals kill pectin. This way the juice does not gel and the fruit releases more fluid.

It is then boiled under vacuum. This means that the temperature is 80 degrees Celsius. In this way the water is extracted from the juice. We get a concentrate.

This concentrate is stored in silos (tanks). In order not to ferment, it is pressed with an inert gas – most often nitrogen. This insulates it from the air and it cannot get sour. It really becomes almost eternal.

The concentrate is sold to the companies producing the final product. It is diluted 1:7, sugar and more additives are added to make it tasty, stabilizers are added so that it does not spoil and so the juice is put in cans.

And let's see briefly: hot pressing kills pectin, vitamins and everything. All that remains is the fructose, from which we accumulate fat in the arteries and between our organs. Also, the chemicals that killed pectin remain. Those artificially added ones, remember? Then boil it again under vacuum. It remains a concentrate of the above. And finally, they add a lot of E's (stabilizers and preservatives), sugar (more fructose) and sell it to us.

No vitamin survives! Nothing useful remains! And even the opposite! And for cover, you buy them for the children and for yourself! Not to mention that every child's birthday has a bottled juice of 30 stotinki delivery price plus pizza!!!

However, there are several manufacturers who claim to apply cold pressing! They are near the towns of Balchik and Yambol. Their production is in glass bottles. The fruits are pressed and must be sealed within 30 minutes. The juice is poured to the neck of the bottle. So, there is no oxygen to oxidize. Half the bottle looks cloudy. This is due to the pectin that survived the pressing. Caps are fitted and the juice is pasteurized by boiling in warm water.

But you will not find vitamins here either. Vitamins live 30 minutes after squeezing the fruit. Even if you make fresh squeeze, the laws are the same. You may have noticed how the color of the juice changes. The same is true with fruit. If you cut an apple, banana or avocado, after a while the cut side is dark and brown. This also happens with juices.

How much fresh juice to drink?

When we make fresh juice, the juicer removes the fibers. If it is fast-moving, it destroys half of the vitamins and useful enzymes contained in the fruit. So we drink only fructose. If it is slow – not with a strainer, but with a screw – it crushes more than it strains. This way the vitamins are preserved. Part of the fiber too. But an apple has the perfect combination of fiber (what feeds us), fructose and glucose. If we squeeze, we remove the fiber (volume) and drink only fructose. We discussed this in previous pages about sugar, fructose is a harmful sugar. It is not absorbed and causes the deposition of fatty toxins in the arteries, blood and lymphatics, liver, heart and between all organs. It becomes internal fat. As are

90% of obese people. And as a bonus, it breaks down collagen and lowers its quality. From there begin problems with joints, bones, sagging skin, wrinkles. In addition to our health, our beauty also goes away.

Therefore, it is best if it is fresh, it should be with the amount of fruit that we would eat if they were not fresh. And yet most useful is to eat the fruit itself. Nature has done everything in a small package wrapped in a peel.

If you make fresh juice from carrots, beets, green vegetables... then do not drink more than 200 ml.

Have a wonderful day, Lovely girl!

Surround yourself with people who will pull you up. Life is full of those who want to drag you down already.

George Clooney

Pigmentation

Do what you can with what you have, wherever you are.

Theodor Roosevelt

Reasons and treatment

Winter is the season when thousands of cosmetic procedures are done for whitening pigmented spots on our sin. Billions are spent on a problem easily regulated with food!

Did I intrigue you?

What exactly is pigmentation?

Pigmentation is increased melanin production in a given area. It is known as a pigment that protects the skin from sunlight. Melanin is formed from two amino acids – phenylalanine and tyrosine in cells called melanocytes. They are located at the base of the skin, eye color, and also form hair shades. In turn, melanocytes are divided into two types. The first takes care of the black and dark brown shades, and the second – the shades from reddish to yellow.

When we have an overproduction of melanin, dark pigment spots appear. When we have reduced production, we have white spots and albinism. The more concentrated the melanocytes, the darker the skin.

Causes of pigmentation

Imagine that your skin is injured, we have acne, we have been in the sun for a long time and it has burned or we have a wound. This is a place where its integrity has been compromised. There begins the formation of young cells. They are low in melanin and unprotected. We expose them to the sun and from this place an impulse is sent to the brain which makes us produce a lot of melanin in a short period of time in order to protect ourselves. Melanocytes in a given area work at full speed and within minutes the area can be pigmented. Indication that they have answered the call.

From my experience and my meeting with clients, the most common causes and injuries are:

Bad wax – when the skin is injured, albeit slightly, pigmentation like a mustache occurs immediately. Many Russian women wax before coming to Bulgaria. The beautician did not tell them that they should put on sunscreen products because they do not have strong sun there and because they did not say that they would go on vacation. It is cold there. Here in the summer, it is 35 degrees and it is easy to burn.

Acne – is injured skin and going out without sunscreen.

Improper cleaning of the face and injury to the turgor of the skin.

Steam bath or sauna in the summer – the skin softens, dehydrates and the next moment we are exposed to the huge heat outside.

What affects the synthesis of melanin?

Age factors – with age, melanocytes stop functioning in the hair first. Over time, throughout the body the skin becomes white as porcelain.

Heredity – appearance of freckles, various spots, etc. For example, white parents may have a dark baby.

UV light, extreme cold or heat – stimulate a rapid and large synthesis of melanin, which colors the skin. Unfortunately, some cells die faster than others and spots appear on the body. The appearance of moles and spots increases.

Improper skin care – very commonly used cosmetics dehydrate the skin. We are not just talking about makeup – powder and foundation. And for daily care – wash gel, milk, tonic, lotion, cream. And how many lotions and shower gels do we use for the body? We will soon talk about harmful substances and how they affect the skin, as well as the greenhouse effect and the damage they cause. Improper care stops the necessary processes and wastes available resources!

Chemical peels and whitening creams – stop the synthesis of melanin, thin the skin and at the first appearance of the sun the spots are present again. Not to mention very often used acids in the summer, which are photosensitive!

Photo and laser procedures – whether it is a program for hair removal, whitening, anti-aging or acne, they often disrupt pigmentation.

Acne and anti-aging creams – many of them are based on vitamin A (and all retinoid derivatives), vitamin E and Q10. Their presence in the cream enhances the pigmentation processes.

Pregnancy – if a pregnant woman puts on a cream like the ones described above, she may get pigmentation in a few minutes. I was one of them myself, from a cream with vitamin A. Separately, we have a hormonal breakdown. The resulting spots are called chloasma. In most cases, this pigmentation occurs on the forehead, cheeks and around the lips.

Vitamin deficiency – if we do not get enough vitamins, magnesium, iron, sulfur, zinc and other vital trace elements in our diet, the skin and tissues do not function properly. If we take too many vitamins A, E, Q10 and folic acid, we internally increase the pigmentation. An indicator of this is the color of the skin. Remember how the skin is a mirror of our inner state?

The color speaks for itself.

Present are chronic diseases of the liver, pancreas and disorders of the heart.

Any stress as well as prolonged use of antibiotics also disrupts melanin synthesis.

Body pigmentation shows the general condition of the body.

We are slaves of our habits. Change your habits and you will change your life.

Robert Kiyosaki

How to Bleach Pigmentation at Home

The most commonly used skin whitening methods are:

Substances containing clarifying components (hydrogen peroxide, mercury, citric acid and salicylic alcohol).

The most effective skin whitening agent is hydroquinone. Unlike the above components, it is very toxic.

Chemical peels, which are divided into deep, superficial and medium. This method of whitening seriously traumatizes the skin, leaving traces on it for a long time. As a rule, redness and swelling after the procedure lasts about a week.

Cryoapplication – this procedure is treatment with liquid nitrogen. Immediately after the procedure, the pigmentation acquires a reddish tinge, after which the surface layer darkens and disappears completely.

The cheapest way to remove pigment spots so far are laser procedures that lead to the destruction of cells containing increased amounts of melanin.

Photoreumatization – the treatment is performed using a high intensity light source that destroys melanin. This method is especially effective for age-related pigmentation.

Did you notice how all of the above are poisonous, toxic or in some way affect the production of melanin, hormones and others. I personally recommend home care to all clients in the last 10 years!

The first option are products, although purchased, based on snail mucus. If the package says 100% mucus, do not take the cream. 100% means hard stone. If the title is untruthful, we don't start well. Read the ingredients! I personally sell and use creams of BAS – Bulgarian Academy of Sciences, made by an associate professor with research over 5 years. The method of extracting the mucus is special and retains over 60% of the useful ingredients. The brand is called Golden-snail and they have an official website.

Live snails! The mucus has a strong lightening effect. I was the first in Bulgaria to offer my clients a procedure with live snails in 2015. If you have a pet snail, it can help. Mine are Achatina (30 cm, carnivorous African snails, but live for a little while if they eat meat, mine did not). Yes, you can put it on your face.

Rubbing the face with cucumber. Cucumber has a strong whitening effect. Rub and stand for 20 minutes every day.

Yogurt – if it's homemade! As a face cream in the evening or as a mask for 20 minutes.

Protein (maybe with aspirin or soda, then burns if there are imperfections, but dries). Mix them to a homogeneous mixture, if it's just protein, beat it. Wash your face, put on the mask and after 20 minutes wash with water. Put on moisturizer.

Rubbing with chamomile tea. Put tea on a cotton swab and apply on the face. Do not wash off, use it as a tonic.

There are many ways! You make the choice!

If you want to succeed, ask yourself those four questions: Why? Why not? Why not me? Why not now?

James Dean

SOS!!! Sweaty Feet!!! SOS!!!

There is hardly anyone who has not experienced this. You go home, take off your shoes and wow... what is this? Sometimes they are just wet, sometimes they are fragrant. I know many people who are worried about taking off their shoes. My kids have been wearing wet socks since they were babies. Why?

Let's start from the inside out

We use cream every night. It contains sulfates, parabens, Vaseline, mineral oils, etc. Substances that make a film over the skin and suffocate it. Imagine wearing gloves all day. Here you will say: "Yes, but I also put on powder." Gloves with talc, without talc... the same. It is no coincidence that in my personal consultations we obligatorily check the composition of the products that my peers use.

Socks. Read the labels. It says "cotton" on the front and 65% cotton, 35% polyester and derivatives on the back. It's the same. Foot bag.

The shoes. Today it is terribly difficult to find nice shoes! By "nice" I don't even mean their appearance. I love sneakers. Of the 50 models of sneakers, only one or two are good. At first glance, they are all made of fabric, right? Yes, but no! Some are pure cotton. Others are of good quality even on the outside, but between the two fabrics (inner and outer) they put an artificial fabric. It rustles slightly. It's like there is cellophane or something rubber between the two layers. One kind will make your feet feel great, they will breathe!!! The other one will be a plastic bag for feet. Leather is also a no.

Even if the shoes are made of genuine leather, many manufacturers add faux leather inside to make them attractive. And what's the difference? Legs, skin, bag and finally – genuine leather. The same thing happens with a nice shoe and a faux sock. Or a nice shoe, a nice sock and for the finish – a suffocating cream or powder. You understand the logic, right?

Sweating is due to hyperfunction of the sweat glands. Medically speaking, hyperhidrosis is divided into primary and secondary. I just opened Google to see what others have written on the subject. Most of the things written are: "The primary is the result of dysfunction of the autonomic nervous system with increased excitability of the sympathetic nervous system." You didn't understand anything, did you?

The autonomic nervous system adapts our body to changes in the environment. Change in temperature and humidity. In short, hotter, more sweat.

Autonomic nervous system – what's on your mind.

Nervous system... If you are tense, you have a lot of stress, the nervous system is like a ping pong ball. It doesn't really understand where it sends the ball. Stress is not just about getting angry and cursing the driver in front of you. Stress is not enough sleep. Stress is bad food. Stress is a rise in glucose and fructose in the body. Stress is blue light. Stress is a rise in adrenaline, bad emotions, cortisol.

It's all connected. There is no way one thing is fine and the other is not.

I wish you a wonderful day!

Feel radiant in your skin!

Hard work is not doing the easy things when you were supposed to.

John Maxwell

Just Like a St. Bernard's Facial Sagging

Do you remember the movie about Beethoven? The dog that had saliva dropping everywhere and drove the man in the family crazy? I laughed out loud at this movie! Unique breed, very loving animals. And if you ask me – very huggable. But I wouldn't want to look like him!

When I started doing cosmetics, I was still a child (18–19 years old). I remember from school how the children invented all sorts of animal nicknames for the teachers: "Sparrow," "Weasel," etc. So, when I saw a sagging face, I remembered Beethoven. And more precisely – St. Bernard. You will often hear me use it in my lectures. At one point, my contour began to sag, and I was 24. And I said to myself, "Ahh no, I don't want my nickname to be St. Bernard!" I began to wonder why it was happening and how to fix it.

The facial contour sags for two reasons

The first is muscle relaxation. How often do you train your facial muscles? So far, I have not done it once! As we want a tight ass, so we have to work for a tight forehead, eye contour and lips. I started training face building.

The second reason – protein. Protein is a building block in the cellular structure of all living organisms. Think of an egg – the white part is protein. And it is twice as much as the other! If the egg is store-bought the white part could be even 3–4 times bigger. Protein helps the human body to renew, grow and develop. Something like a shopping bag. We arrive home and start: the apples in the fruit cupboard, the eggs on the refrigerator door, the meat in the fridge, etc. Protein is divided into other constituent units, without which we cannot survive! One of them is amino acids.

If protein is missing or the amounts are reduced, our body will react with slow growth, loss of muscle and organ mass, accompanied by disease. I can give my younger daughter as a development example. She is a protein type and eats three times more meat than her sister, who is a carbohydrate type. When one was 2 and a half years old, the other was 4 and 2 months old, but they wore the same size shoes and clothes!

There is a second option: eating excessive amounts of protein for long periods of time. Impaired kidney and liver function. This leads to various diseases and shortens life. Example: achatinas. These are African snails that grow up to 30 cm long. I was raising them for 5 years. They can be carnivorous or herbivorous. If they eat only grass, they grow at a normal rate and live about 8 years. If they eat meat, dog or cat food – they grow for days instead of years!

And now – do you remember the information about collagen? Thirty-three percent of the proteins in our body are collagen. Bone, muscles, tendons and 75% of the skin are made of collagen. What's in our face? Muscle and skin! What happens when there is little protein? Sagging! What breaks down quality collagen? Mainly sugar (especially fructose) and white flour. What makes us swell and stretch our skin? Refined salt, white flour, sugar and pasteurized dairy products. Swelling equals stretching. You can't stretch skin all the time and want it to tighten. **You have to stop stretching it first and then tighten it!**

Protein, in particular collagen, gives density, structure and elasticity! Missing collagen intake? Or have we lowered the quality from a lot of sugar and harmful substances? The contour of the face is sagging.

Learn to recognize the red lights on the body panel. The fact that the contour is sagging is your least problem! The real problems are inside you, hidden from your eyes.

Now take a mirror and look at yourself: what is your face like? Does it have pigmentation, pimples, sagging, oily skin?

Now see where exactly! Repair the reason we talked about and be beautiful and irresistible! But above all healthy! **Act**! And if you start thinking, "But I'm 56," stop that thought! Age doesn't matter! I'm sure you're keeping something from your childhood that looks the same as when it was given to you! Metabolic age (the years tissues and organs work according to) and your real age have nothing in common! I'm 30 calendar years old. My body works like a 14-year-old. And it wasn't always like that!

You will never be too old to set a new goal and dream of something new.

Clive Staples Lewis

Gold in a Bottle for Only 1.65 Leva

Have you heard of castor oil? Yes, the one in the pharmacies, in brown bottles for 1.65 leva, and in some places for 1.20 leva. The same! To me, it's like gold in a bottle. This is one of those little bottles and jars that must be in the closet of every woman who cares about her beauty! Why?

Because it is priceless!

And at the same time very underestimated! I love simple things. They work many times more than complex mixtures.

I will try to tell you how briefly!

Its effect on the skin is highly moisturizing and antibacterial. Helps with oily skin, dry skin, dehydration, sunburn, stretch marks, acne, warts, keratoses, fungal infections, fungal and bacterial infections. It can be used in many ways.

As a cleaning agent – apply to the face and rub it in. Then wash. If a specific area is affected (acne, infection, etc.), apply, leave for an hour and wash off or sleep with it. If the area is seriously affected, it is good to apply twice a day. Because it shines, in the morning we can wash it with warm water or mix it with our cream.

Think of all those small, fine lines and wrinkles all over your face and especially those around your eyes.

They annoy you, don't they?

Most often they are due to dehydration in the face. Put caster oil on to your face every night for 2–3 weeks instead of face cream. You can also add it to your cream. Castor oil penetrates deeply and helps stimulate elastin and collagen. The skin becomes thicker and firmer. And here you have a bonus! Eyelashes and eyebrows become thick, black and shiny in 2 weeks, and for two more they become long and voluminous.

The contained castor acid helps to regenerate the skin by slightly exfoliating. And in the presence of acne, this acid is like an antiseptic. But unlike anti-acne drugs, it does not dry the skin.

Scars (from acne or old pimples) and stretch marks recover very quickly. Thanks to the beneficial fatty acids, the skin regenerates, dry spots disappear. Thus, there is no danger of pigmentation.

The same fatty acids help whiten the skin. The pigment spots become much paler, until finally, all the bumps, freckles and pigmentation processes simply disappear.

Castor oil is ideal for first aid (scratches, injuries, wounds). It accelerates the healing process and has antibacterial action.

There's a catch here! If the face is prone to hair, put only on the problematic areas! I think you remember why.

And now about the hair and the scalp:

We have already mentioned the plus for eyelashes and eyebrows.

Castor oil stimulates hair growth! It becomes thick and dense, shiny and hydrated, lively and elastic. We forget about split ends. My shampoo is hand-made in Sofia by the "Soap Workshop" and costs 6 leva for 220 ml. It contains castor oil. I take a bath and my hair becomes dry with volume and at the same time I feel how greasy it is inside. The first time I thought I hadn't washed it well. I had to wash it again, but I fell asleep and went to bed. The next day my hair had absorbed the fat. Every day instead of my hair getting oilier, it got prettier. You can add oil to your shampoo in the same way. But you have to break it down very well! The oil is rich in omega 3, 6 and 9 fatty acids, which nourish and help retain moisture in the hair and scalp. Contains vitamin E, proteins and minerals that give density and strength. The hair becomes thick and dense. Forget about thin ends and breakage.

The antibacterial action helps with dandruff. Put a little oil on your hands and rub into the scalp. Stand like this for 20 minutes to an hour and wash. This oil is very difficult to wash if it is a concentrate, so use a delicate amount. If you have split ends, put very little on the tips, sleep like that or stand for at least 20 minutes and wash. You will be surprised by the result.

And hair loss is just a memory!

Nails:

Do you have brittle and soft nails? Smear them every night and after two weeks write me a comment on "what happened."

And finally, how it affects the body:

Castor oil effectively cures tapeworm, a scientifically proven fact!

In case of constipation or difficult defecation, take 1 tsp. for 2–3 days and the problem disappears; it facilitates the work of the gastrointestinal tract and cleanses the colon.

In joint pain and arthritis it has an analgesic and anti-inflammatory effect. Apply directly to the affected area and rub.

Enhances lymphatic drainage. Castor oil helps the lymph to move faster. And from previous articles you already know how important that is!

After reading this, I am sure that if you pass a pharmacy, you will buy it. And from today this will be one of the things you will always have on your shelf.

Smiling day, Wonderful!!! Be feminine and irresistible! Feel unsurpassed in your skin!

I dare you! Today you have to catch the eye of at least three strangers and smile at them! You will be surprised how happy this will make you feel!

The ship is safe in the port but it is not built for that.

Grace Hopper

The Secret of Wax

Do you wax? I will tell you a secret now!

All bacteria, candida and infections live in the wax – from candida to sexually transmitted diseases. How did I find this out? As I worked. I opened a new wax package, did intimate hair removal, my next client is fine and boom – the next day she is not. By "clients" I mean my relatives and friends who I know have no problems! One time, a second... tenth, twentieth. And we noticed it.

I'll tell you here that I don't do it anymore. Because I know that your brain will keep repeating to you that it is an advertisement!

After a while I started doing individual waxing. I bought small tin cans. I took two hotplates. One for the big wax mask with the box, the other so I can put the little dose inside the tin can.

What does it spare for us? All those pimples and subcutaneous hairs! When there is a bacterium, it enters through the injured skin where the hair is removed. It's an infection! From there, the skin becomes rough. Through it, the new hair cannot come out. It becomes subcutaneous. When I had a new client, in two months all these problems disappeared.

Have you ever waxed your moustache and then got pimples? What does bulk waxing do? Whatever was on the client, goes in the box. Not to mention that many beauticians use a metal spatula and do not change it at all. I had ladies who removed the hair on their entire face every 6 months. And they didn't have a single pimple! They couldn't wait to do it, because it's like peeling and skin renewal! I'm not saying to wax your face! When you start, more hairs start to grow!

And here I will say a few things about depilators. This is a packet with a lot of chemicals! These chemicals penetrate your skin and cause a lot of different damage. The substances do not stay in one place but are distributed throughout the body. It is only a matter of time before it harms you.

Take care of yourself! A smiling day, Irresistible!

Belt – Bad Or...?

Road to nowhere is paved with excuses.

Mark Bell

Hello.

Again, the gym was filled with new faces and I remembered how many of them train with belts. Every day I repeat the same thing like a gramophone record. So, I decided to share it with you.

Why do we wear a belt during training? If you are a woman, it is because you want to lose weight. You sweat more. And why don't you sweat without a belt? Do you drink water? Are you standing properly on the bike or in your sport? This means the middle finger is forward, ankle, knee, pelvis is in one line. The abdomen is inwards. The back is straight and levelled. Shoulders back. Chin at 90 degrees from the neck. If you don't drink water, if you don't stand properly and if you don't do as your coach tells you... forget to sweat.

The second reason you share with me is, "otherwise my lower back hurts." Yes, because you twist it. You arch it and burden it. The idea of exercising is to learn how to tighten, to strengthen the lower abdominal wall! It does not strengthen with pushups! Many people in the gym train, stand on their elbows on a device, tighten their arms, relax on their shoulders (shoulders are very much up) and lift the legs. Then you still do not train what you have to! You just further ruin your lower back, the shoulders go upwards and you start to hunch in your everyday life. The neck shortens.

Why do men wear belts? You've seen them lift weights. Have you seen a weightlifter without a belly? It is not important for them to have a tight abdomen. It is important that their legs and arms have the strength to push. Look at them. If they lift the weight, their back becomes C-shaped. All the tension is in the spine. Imagine 10 cubes with an elastic band in the middle. If they are on top of each other everything is okay. But if you make a circle with them... it's not like that anymore. The rubber band thins, the cubes wear out. Well, this is your spine. And these are your tendons and bone marrow.

Let's see what actually happens

We have a natural belt. It holds the whole structure of the body. This is our core. It consists of the lower abdominal wall, upper abdominal wall, waist and part of the diaphragm. Draw a circle. Its contour is you, seen from above. On one side is the abdomen, on the other is the waist. Your spine is in the contour, in the back. It is gripped and stands firmly. It can't move chaotically! The belt supports it. Now draw another, larger circle over this one. This is a belt you wear for training. It tightens the bottom and our inner belt doesn't need to work. It relaxes. The spine is not in the grip. It can move wherever it wants. The tendons stretch. When you put on a plaster, what happens? When you remove the plaster, are you healthier? The muscle seems to have atrophied and is weaker. Yes, right?

All the tension goes to the spine. You don't tighten. You do not lose weight. You have no result. You're just sweating!

Today, when I make someone breathe properly, they feel dizzy. We have forgotten to breathe because we are hunched over which automatically shuts off a strong diaphragm. It is trained only by breathing. Belly? Many have an upper abdominal wall – six pack. I admit it. But too tight and too short. It loses its elasticity. From there, the lower back moves forward in a C-shape. It is weak and stretched. It is tired of the upper abdominal wall pulling it constantly. Lower abdominal wall? Do you have a belly? This means you do not have a lower abdominal wall. It is from the triangle (inclusive) to the navel.

Exercise without a belt! Otherwise, you are not doing yourself a favor. What you can do yourself, no one else can!

Strengthen the lower abdominal wall. Do not do complicated exercises. Straighten up. Strengthen your core! It defines you. It determines your quality of life. It determines whether you will hurt your back while lifting children, changing the sheets or having sex.

Up to you!

Life is a great big canvas, and you should throw all the paint on it you can.

Danny Kaye

Varicose Veins:
Why? Prevention and Treatment!

A journey of a thousand miles begins with a single step.

Lao Tzu

What are varicose veins? Imagine a river flowing unhindered. Its end flows into its beginning. Something like a circle. The current is strong and attracts all the garbage that falls into it to the end (kidneys). One day a tree falls. Little by little in this place the river accumulates garbage and becomes a dam. The load there is great and it starts making its way around the dam. The trough dilates (in this area we begin to accumulate body fat) and blood vessels suffer from pressure.

No matter the dam, it affects everything equally – the river becomes slow in places, fast in places. The main reasons for the appearance of the dam are:

1. Distortions – from flat feet, contraction or opening of the knees, displaced pelvis forward or backward through the spine to the head. Just because we have a varicose vein behind the knee doesn't mean the source of the problem is the knee!

2. Sitting with crossed legs – the one on top is squeezing the veins. We don't have to numb our toes to believe it. A large amount of fluid wants to pass through the gap. Imagine holding a balloon. Have you noticed how it doesn't crack, but becomes translucent in the stretched place? And after you let it go, it stays somehow more swollen? The lower leg has lymph pressure. It cannot clear and cellulite begins to appear above the knee.

Do your experiment! When it's warm outside, look at the legs of the women around you. One leg always has more cellulite than the other above the knee, and the other has more varicose veins behind the knee than the first!

3. Improper sleeping position – if we sleep in the fetal position and intertwine our legs with our partner, we apply the same pressure. I will not comment on the lack of nutrients and the impossibility of clearing waste products. We have already talked about it. If the veins have started to stretch in this area, you will feel a slight pulsation in a given place, as if your heart is beating from there.

4. Wrongly applied anti-cellulite procedures – incorrect anti-cellulite massage! Wrongly applied pressure therapy and lymphatic drainage! Both the device and the specialist are very important here!

5. Thermal products – heating products are not applied where there are superficial veins. As for the knee.

6. Improper breathing – nowadays we all breathe very shallowly. We stand hunched over at work, in the car, we sleep bent, we train without thinking about when we inhale and exhale. Little by little the liver is crushed. We get used to breathing with our upper part. To look good, we put on tight bras. We use pants that press our waist, we swallow the stomach artificially, not knowing how to breathe! Proper breathing has a straight spine and breathes sideways – like the gills of a fish. Oxygen deficiency prevents very important processes that release the hormones responsible for the elasticity of blood and lymph vessels in our body. Which also affect our memory and concentration! Not to mention all the risks of heart disease – heart attack, stroke, etc. Oxygen is also needed for tissue regeneration. No oxygen – no regeneration and elasticity.

We don't have to wait to get varicose veins! Skin color alone shows if we have oxygen! Our memory! If we breathe heavily! All these are indications that something will happen soon.

How to prevent it and how to treat it?

1. Laser – eliminates the problem, closes the main highway and all the load goes to the secondary roads. Sooner or later, everything happens again.
2. Cardio training – teaches us to breathe. We saturate with oxygen. And all the processes start working.
3. We sleep properly! On the back. This is how we straighten the spine. In the beginning it will hurt where we have distortions. And after a month or two it disappears. We open all the lymph and blood channels and everything starts to spin quickly.
4. We do not sit cross-legged. Sit at the end of the chair, keep your spine straight, step on a full foot and make sure that your thighs are not pinched at the bottom of the chair as soon as you lower your knees.
5. Cosmetics – you can use grape seed oil every day on the problem area.
6. Learn to breathe. There is only one exercise for the muscles in the diaphragm located on the inside of the ribs. If you activate them, you will learn to breathe with your ribs opening to the side with a swallowed belly (indicating that you keep the muscles active and the body stable)!

At SEMMA trainings I cured more than one or two from varicose veins. I forgot about the pain behind my knee. At 20, I had cellulite. To get rid of it, I went to pressure therapy which was given to me with a medical device from a rehabilitator. The result was varicose veins. After the first pregnancy, the situation became tragic. I couldn't bend my legs. My veins hurt 24 hours a day. Everything cleared for a month. SEMMA is corrective gymnastics on a spinning wheel and includes breathing techniques that have won a place in the Guinness Book of Records. What is happening? I breathe – I saturate with oxygen. I have movement – I carry it around.

If you have varicose veins, start thinking about how to help yourself. If you don't, make sure it stays that way. If you don't think you can do it alone, welcome to training. Tell me that's your goal. Train with me for a month. And if you still have varicose veins, I'll give you your money back.

If you want others to believe in you, you need to believe in yourself first!

Unknown

How to Choose a Cutting Board

There is hardly a day when we do not use a cutting board! Different types are available on the market: wooden, plastic, ceramic and glass.

But how does it affect our body?

The most common are bamboo and wooden cutting boards. Unfortunately, every time you cut on it, the wooden surface is injured. Particles of the food we cut are inserted into the barely noticeable incisions. In the presence of juice, it absorbs into the board. If we wash it with detergent, it also gets absorbed. All this is impossible to wash out 100%. Thus, the surface becomes an ideal environment for the development of all forms of life that we cannot see with the naked eye. The moisture that is retained in the board and the putrefactive processes that we do not see, in addition to microscopic food particles, become an ideal breeding ground for all kinds of pathogens. If detergents are used, even washing detergent, it penetrates with the water into the wooden surface. In the next cut, we cut from the tree and consume it with food.

All this can cause skin problems such as acne, pigmentation, dry skin and eczema. Also, serious health problems with the digestive tract, cardiovascular system, urinary system, nerves, irritability, frequent illness, asthma and much more. Depending on the bacterial flora that has developed, there are different consequences. If you still want to cut on a wooden board, look for unglued. The adhesives used are often toxic, and when cut, we consume them with food.

Recently, plastic boards have become popular. If they are made of plastic that does not scratch or emit toxic substances, they are a good solution. But they are rarely found because they are expensive, and many consumers do not know and do not look for the difference. In over 90% of cases, the boards are scratched and we take the food from the toxic plastic. And in the scratch things are just the same as with the wood.

I only use glass and ceramic boards. Again, they are heat resistant, but do not scratch. They can be washed with detergents under running water as well as in a dishwasher. They do not need to be replaced because they are do not deteriorate. And last but not least, they are very beautiful. For me, they are like a picture that gives me a mood, leaning on the counter. I have one big and one small. My little one is for quick work. And my big one is for meat, fish, tomatoes and all kinds of runny things. Why are there two? Because the big one is heavier and the small one is more comfortable. Because the big one doesn't spill on the table and counter.

I personally value my health! And I am happy when something so small helps me.

What about you?

Our fate is formed by those little invisible decisions that we make 100 times a day.

Anthony Robbins

PS. Metal knives oxidize when being used. I recommend a 100% ceramic knife.

Heal Stretch Marks

I don't know if there is a woman who doesn't care about this issue!?! For the 8 years I worked with cosmetics and anti-cellulite treatments, I tried every expensive brand I came across that had anti-stretch mark therapies. Result: None! Until a year ago I tried something quite by accident and healed my own – at home.

But let's start from the beginning. What are stretch marks? An indication that we are missing something. There are several times when stretch marks appear – adolescence, pregnancy, weight loss and weight gain, endocrine diseases and long-term glucocorticoid treatment. In the last two, stretch marks are all over the body, even on the face! The rest are on the thighs, buttocks, hips, chest, arms. Stretch marks can appear when exposed to the sun if the skin is very dry! Imagine the sea, salt water, sun and you on the beach. Sounds wonderful! If the skin has missing or delayed regeneration processes, it will shrink like a garment in the dryer that should not have been there.

Stages:

First stage – pink stretch marks, which may slightly itch. The skin around them looks scalded.

Second stage – stretch marks grow in width and length, it is possible to become very red.

Third stage – their color changes to milky white or grayish, it is possible that they take on irregular shapes, and their roughness disappears. This is due to their sealing in the skin as a scar. We are already in the stage of old stretch marks.

What's wrong and when do they appear?

In the case of poor nutrition. A large percentage of our food is something like a carton. It satisfies us but has zero value! And the other percentage of consumption of the average citizen is a box sprinkled with many harmful toxic and carcinogenic substances. They unbalance the production of important hormones, lower the quality of collagen and elastin (collagen is a building block in our body), cause infections and a host of other diseases. Adherence to meaningless diets such as "eat only this," "drink only water," "live on yogurt and oatmeal" and all other restrictions also cause the above.

The low quality of collagen, its reduced synthesis and the substances that stimulate its production are of the greatest importance for the appearance of stretch marks.

Prevention of stretch marks:

Eat well. Eat vegetables, fruits, meat, healthy fats. Drink 0. 033 liters of water per kilogram. If you drink coffee, green tea or other dehydrating drinks, add 0.500 liters on top. Do not eat white sugar, refined salt, white flour, colorants and preservatives. Increase your intake of vitamins A and C. Remember what we talked about in the article about the hands. The face is the tab with lights, you just have to read the instructions. Add to your diet what your skin wants! Apply natural oils. Read the packaging and make sure there are no parabens, SLS, mineral oils and all harmful substances. During pregnancy, apply from the first month before you swell. It takes skin 3 months to soak in!

Treatment:

I had been eating well for several years, but it wasn't enough. My stretch marks are from high school – white as snowflakes. I have tried anti-cellulite and all sorts of procedures to reduce it. The effect is short. They smooth out, but they are still visible. I stopped the procedures and again... they disappeared after a little home therapy.

1. Once or twice a week I make juice from orange, lemon, celery, beets, carrots, apples, add parsley or spinach. I drink the juice and rub the bran into my body for about 10 minutes. Here the important thing is the vitamins that

we drink and that we take through the skin! Therefore, the fruits may be different each time. Fundamental, are carrots (vitamin A) and citrus (vitamin C)! After rubbing, wash only with water! No detergent!

2. After this shower I put natural collagen. Slightly dry and apply to damp skin all over the body. In this way cellulite is reduced and taken directly from the skin. I use natural Polish live collagen. There is only collagen and water in the bottle. Here I will give you a gift. You can order it with a discount from SEMMA.BG. Just send a photo of you with this book at office@semma.bg. I use Silver. There are different models.

3. Two or 3 times a week (on other days!) I use cocoa butter! I combined it with going to the seaside. I applied butter on the beach and after we got home, I washed only with water, without shower gel.

For a month, all the stretch marks were a memory, and my skin looked like it was on the cover of a magazine, processed in Photoshop!

Act! No matter how old you are, you deserve to feel like a queen in your skin!

You learn fastest in 3 cases: up to 7 years of age, at the treadmill or when life pushes you in the corner.

Steven Covey

Hazardous Components in Cosmetics

Oil-based creams cover the skin like stretch film. They suffocate it like a "greenhouse effect," deprive it of a constant flow of oxygen and block many of its secretory functions (this is where the appearance of inflammation and blackheads begins). The skin is soaked with water and the body forbids moisturizing as unnecessary. If you put a plastic bag on your head for 24 hours, when you breathe, everything will be filled with drops of water. You feel like you are suffocating. As a result, the skin dries out or artificially begins to become oily and has enlarged pores. Let's see which products cause it.

Technical oils:

Mineral oil

Petrolatum

Paraffinum liquidum

Dioxine – so far, all cause breast cancer.

And also:

SLS sSodium lauryl sulfate) and its derivatives (ammonium lauryl sulfate, ammonium lauryl sulfate, sodium lauryl sulfate, TEA lauryl sulfate, TEA lauryl sulfate) – are available in all foaming products – toothpastes, soaps, shower gels, etc. Aggressive foaming agents that disrupt the natural pH of the skin are highly carcinogenic, form carcinogenic dioxins and nitrates that accumulate in tissues and are toxic in large doses. Penetrating into the body, SLS accumulates in the tissues of the eyes, brain, liver. They may cause hair loss and dandruff. We will talk about it separately.

Silicones (dimethicone, amodimethicone and all others ending in -cone) – create an indelible layer of stretch film, stopping the penetration of nutrients.

Phthalates – cause abnormalities in the body, endocrine disorders. Two of them, regularly used in cosmetics – dibutyl and diethylhexyl – are banned in EU countries. Diethylphthalate and dimethylphthalate are most common in perfumes, mousses, hair gels and nail polishes. They have a strong harmful effect on DNA. If a woman has used phthalate cosmetics during pregnancy, it can adversely affect the fetus if the child is male. These chemicals block the processes that regulate male sex hormones – androgens. This can lead to impotency and infertility.

Parabens (propylparaben, methylparaben, butylparaben, ethylparaben, phenoxyethanol) – highly toxic substances, preservatives that accumulate in the body and cause hormonal disorders.

TEA, DEA (triethanolamine, diethanolamine) – toxic, carcinogenic substances.

Propylene glycol (polypropylene glycol), Polyethylene glycol (polyethylene glycol or antifreeze) – toxic, carcinogenic substances. They cause changes in the liver and damage the kidneys.

Formaldehyde, toluene – toxic, carcinogenic substances.

Mercury (thimerosal) – a strong neurotoxin that affects the functions of the brain and nervous system. Possible human carcinogen and toxin affecting human reproduction and development. It is found in some eye drops, mascaras and creams.

Triclosan – is often used as an antibacterial agent in the production of soap, lotions, deodorants, shower gels, creams toothpastes. It has a detrimental effect on the endocrine system, more precisely it affects the thyroid gland. If combined with chlorine, the formation of chloroform is possible, which is possibly a carcinogen.

Placenta – may confuse human hormonal function and cause serious health problems (breast cancer, for example).

Lead Acetate – affects reproduction and development. It is banned for use in cosmetics in the EU. Found in some cleansing creams and hair dyes.

Hydroquinone – a possible carcinogen and possible neurotoxin, makes the skin sensitive. It can also cause a skin condition called ochronosis (black and blue patches on the skin). It has a pronounced depigmenting effect. It is most often found in whitening creams.

Or in other words, why can't we do without our precious cream and buy another box before the old one runs out? We apply tons of cream and makeup, and the skin underneath feels dry. For the same reason, over 95% of clients who come to me for cosmetic procedures think they have oily skin and try to dry it. They actually have dry skin that produces sebum quickly because it is used to drying it out. But we will talk more about this in my next book.

Be careful what you use! We take many more substances through the skin than through the mouth. This is especially dangerous for young children, who in the twenty-first century are in the habit of bathing and smearing on thousands of products every day!

Smiling day, Fairy!

Ema

Fruit Temptation

Do you like the aroma of fruit? I loved my shower gel smelling delicious. I couldn't wait to finish it to get a new scent. Banana, strawberry, melon, orange or other citrus, watermelon... It's as if I wash my body and awaken my senses. This sounds like a gum advertisement.

And a fact! Your sense of smell has the ability to change your hormones. When a certain aroma is felt, the body reacts. Why do some scents excite you, others soothe you, still others make you nervous? Why does everyone like a different scent? This is the reason why there are so many variations of a product with 50 flavors and aromas. Everyone wants to feel different, so they want a different scent.

In the past, this has been achieved with oils. Now I will tell you my secret for concentration. I do not use perfumes. If there is a day when I want to concentrate as if I had 5 coffees, my brain works like high-speed internet – I use oil! A drop of lemongrass distributed between my wrists and behind my ears works wonders! Did you go to the NESEMINAR 2017? Yuli invited me to share what I had achieved, thanks to his motivation. I spoke in front of 2,500 people, my thoughts flowed smoothly, I made the audience laugh and clap more than once. Well – I was on lemongrass. I got up at 04:00 because Doni wanted to be sure we wouldn't be late. I didn't want to stress her out and we left early. I had 4 boiled eggs for breakfast in the car at 08:00. I usually eat every four hours. On that day during the breaks, I couldn't keep quiet because everyone was asking me something. They took about 400 business cards and asked me about 2,000 questions. I managed to leave at 21:30 and was in Burgas at 00:40. And I was 100% productive.

The winter fairy tale – the same! Master classes – the same! Some 16 hours in which you give your best and you are here and now without 10 seconds of distraction! This is the lemongrass. It awakens your senses!

If you want to sleep or calm down, your oil is lavender.

Oils change your perceptions and stimulate the synthesis of certain hormones. The Greeks lubricated their hair with oils. The idea was to hide the aroma from the lack of a bath. But it has subsequently become a way of influencing the body and others. Why do we use aroma oils when meditating? Why are there Aromatherapies in every spa? Impact! Influence on emotions! With a certain oil you can provoke emotion. Today, people are very difficult to control. We are constantly experiencing emotions, and we do not know how to provoke them ourselves. We have forgotten that body positions determine how we feel.

Do you remember the information about harmful substances? Now I will reveal another trick.

Shower gel dries your skin. We absorb all harmful substances through the skin. We're getting toxic. What would you say if every shower made you feel ecstatic with pleasure and had the aroma of chocolate, strawberry, melon, watermelon, banana, lemon or another favorite flavor? It will cost you pennies! And at the same time, you will saturate your skin with vitamins. Useful and enjoyable!

How?

I took 2 strawberries. I crushed a half between my fingers and slowly rubbed my face. I stayed like this for 20 minutes. Instead of shower gel I crushed the other halves and put them on my body. I washed with water and had the aroma of fresh strawberries all day with me!

The acid in the fruit regenerates the skin, gives shine, saturates with vitamins, removes subcutaneous hairs, removes stretch marks and there are many other benefits that you can see for yourself! Today I made a hair mask with castor oil. It's 6:30 in the morning and it has already soaked up. In the blender I mixed 1/2 banana, 1 egg yolk, 1 tsp. nutritional yeast and made a hair mask. I smeared the same on my face. If I didn't take a bath with my hair the night before the shower, I would just rub my face with a banana. I go all over my body with the rest of the mask, or just a little banana.

The summer with watermelon is an indescribable feeling! With a melon or cucumber – the freshness is 100%!

Do you like chocolate? I really like to make chocolate masks. It is a very strong antioxidant. I also use it for shower gel. But cosmetic chocolate. Every brand has one. It is hard. Melt it in and you're done.

In this case, the need for products to lubricate your skin after a bath disappears! The skin does not dry out. If it still stretches, smear it with cocoa butter. What you eat! And not cosmetically! You want a coconut flavor – coconut oil! Put only what you would eat on the skin!

What shower gels give you is 0.01% of what fruit concentrate gives you. Crazy money is given for peelings with fruit acids. And why not turn them into a ritual of pleasure and bliss every day?

The joy of life is in the little things! In simple things! In the things we do routinely every day! The children are happy that they managed to tie their shoes! How they jumped over the puddle! That they chose socks!

Give yourself emotion! Give yourself mood!

I wish you an unforgettable and fresh day!

May it be as wonderful as you are!

The only man who makes no mistakes is the man who never does anything. Do not be afraid to make mistakes providing you do not make the same one twice.

Theodore Roosevelt

I Forgot!

Do you know people who "will forget their head somewhere and will not notice"!

Yes, I was talking about you.

And here we do not comment on chronic diseases, nor in the case where we work in 10 places and forget things, we empty the glass. We are talking about the case in which we are to blame!

There are several ways we can influence this and they are interconnected!

1. Water – 74 to 90% of our brain is water. How much water do you drink per day? Imagine a jellyfish left in the sun without water.

   Hmmm yeah.... this also happens to our brain when we are dehydrated. Every day the water norm is 0.033 liters per kilogram. If we drink coffee or other dehydrator plus another 0.5 liters per cup taken. The first dehydration in our body occurs in the brain. We begin to squat, crush the lungs and organs, apply additional internal pressure. Not to mention that by moving forward we increase the weight of the body many times over.

   The solution is to drink water!

2. Sleep position – If we sleep with a pillow, we pinch the only large arteries in the neck that should feed the brain, skin, hair and everything on our head. We wake up with swelling and puffiness, the lymph has not done its job and has not cleared. Don't think you're puffy just under your eyes.

   You can't stretch and shrink your skin, tissue and brain several times a day and expect to have memory and beauty...

   The solution is to sleep on your back, without a pillow.

3. Poor blood circulation – if you have no movement, sit for many hours at work, sleep all curled up, sit cross-legged or "Turkish style" and a bunch of strange poses, then you slow down the flow of the river that flows inside you. And from a raging river in high tide season, there is a small stream in the middle of the land.

   The solution is to think how you sleep, how you sit; think what you do!

4. Lack of nutrients – the quality of our food determines our quality of life! It determines who we are: the curve "permanently on her period," distracted, party girl, alcoholic, always smiling, mother-in-law, etc. If your food lacks quality, negative radicals and value... then your life will be a cycle of fatigue, crookedness, and forgetfulness.

   The solution is to increase your intake of fruits and vegetables. Cut down on sweets, chips, fried foods and anything you think is harmful (except butter and animal fats, which are not harmful but help you). You can add ginkgo biloba, baobab and other foods that open the circulatory system and improve irrigation, as I do. I choose only crushed herbs that I put directly into my smoothie.

5. Lack of muscle tone – when we have weak muscle tone, there is nothing to help the blood vessels carry nutrients, and the lymph to dispose of garbage. The river slows down again. It's just waiting for gravity to work – well, okay, but it just pulls down...

   The solution is to move!

6. Lack of oxygen –From pinching of the arteries, poor blood circulation, lack of muscle tone and improper breathing, we fall into oxygen deficiency. Oxygen is like an additive in the blood that raises the quality of all processes in it. Something like gas and Vpower 100 octane with additive. There is a difference, isn't there? In the absence of oxygen,

blood vessels lose elasticity. They lose their ability to stretch and contract. So, it is very difficult for us in the warm, and very cold in the cold. Varicose veins begin to appear, not only on the legs. There is something like the red light on the dashboard that makes us think.

The solution is to breathe sideways and open the diaphragm like the gills of a fish. At the beginning of oversaturation, you will feel dizzy, but this is an indication that you are breathing for the first time!

7. Energy saving – the less you use, the less you produce! Finally, you fall into emergency mode! Think about how many people around you look in this state, as if on autopilot. This is not how we live; this is how we simply exist!

The solution is to spend more energy and you will produce more energy! Demand determines supply!

There are no people who are just born distracted! This is another excuse for the brain to be right. It is no coincidence that in SEMMA we breathe according to certain methods! When you train and see varicose veins disappear... priceless! Change the above 7 things and you will remember everything in detail!

And here I come to ask you: do you notice how everything is connected? Each chapter of this book leads to another 4–5. Everything is like a big network and you can't have a small problem. Something small stops the work of the entire network!

When you introduce something new, be ready to be called crazy.

Larry Ellison

Believe you can and you are already half way through.

Theodor Roosevelt

Gluten Mania

Have you heard of gluten?

Have you heard of harmful substances in food?

Have you heard of plant proteins?

More and more often I see and hear people who have decided to eat "healthy." To order and buy gluten-free foods. Let's see what kind of animal is this? For some, it is quality food, for others it is class and mania. For others, however, it is something they know is harmful and they avoid, but do not know why.

You can't help but hear an advertisement or notice the inscriptions on the packaging – Gluten free. The word "glue" comes from the English language. The word speaks for itself. Something that sticks to us. It is this "glue" that sticks to the lining of the small intestine and forms inflammation. No, don't stop, wait, there's more.

I will surprise you even more with the fact that gluten is a vegetable protein! Yes exactly! You already know that there are different metabolic types – protein, carbohydrate and mixed, but they all eat protein! The difference is that some absorb vegetable protein better, others, animal protein. Gluten is composed of gliadin and glutenin, forming a protein mixture. In fact, intolerance to this mixture is called a gluten allergy. The medical word for this is celiac disease.

If you type "diet" into the search engine you get over 1,000,000 different offers. Half of them are gluten free!

Does it make sense to avoid it? Only if you can't process it.

But how did such harmful foods suddenly come out? So many diets have been created? Is this fashion? Or do people really realize what's going on?

I do a lot of diets and I don't think people realize that yet. At least not all. If you've come this far with reading, you're the type who reads the lowercase letters on food labels. The guy who's not obsessed with thinking about what to eat. And I will not use "healthy," because the meaning of this word has long been distorted. I would say quality and value!

Let me continue with the gluten. Today, in order for cereals to be more resilient to harsh conditions, they are genetically modified. However, this destroys us! Many materials and articles have been written on this topic.

I will give you examples of foods that contain gluten:

cereals and grains (wheat, rye, barley, wheat, oats, graham, einkorn),As well as derivatives – flour, pasta, macaroni, starch, barley,sausages,

ice cream,

chocolate, caramel,

fried foods (breaded), croutons,

muesli and roasted nuts,

ground spices (curry, turmeric, paprika, cinnamon),

soy sauce,

baking powder and sweeteners,

beer,

ketchup, mustard and ready-made sauces and

surprise! – coffee!

It's very easy – read the label! It says everything, unless it's a trick for an easy sale and it says "gluten free," when in fact it has it. Then it would be much harder to understand the truth. Also, in order to sell their goods, they include the name of gluten with different names such as avena saliva (oat) kernel flour, cyclodextrin, dextrin, dextrin palmitate, hydrolyzed malt extract, hydrolyzed oat flour, hydrolyzed vegetable, protein, hydrolyzed wheat flour, hydrolyzed wheat gluten, hydrolyzed, wheat protein, hydrolyzed wheat protein / PVP crosspolymer, hydrolyzed wheat starch, secale cereale (rye) seed flour, triticum, vulgare (wheat) germ extract, triticum vulgare (wheat) germ oil, triticum vulgare (wheat) gluten, triticum vulgare (wheat) starch, wheat, amino acids, wheat germ glycerides, wheat germamidopropalkonium, chloride, wheat protein, wheatgermamidopropyl ethyldimonium, ethosulfate, yeast extract.

Better light a small candle than curse the darkness.

Chinese proverb

Hazardous Components

I will not waste your time with empty letters and lines. I will give you an example with some ingredients and what they cause. You decide if you will check the labels for their presence.

E200 - Sorbic acid – whether it is obtained from bones or synthesized from chestnut, its presence may cause skin irritation.

E210 - Benzoic acid – phenylcarboxylic acid. It is added to alcoholic products, cheeses, spices, frozen foods, in cosmetics and pharmaceutical products and many others. May cause asthma, especially with steroid addicts. It may interact with sulfur bisulfite (222), which may lead to hyperactivity in children.

E211 Sodium benzoate – is used as an antiseptic, food preservative and flavor masking agent. Orange juices contain a high amount, up to 25 mg per 250 ml. It is also found in dairy and meat products, in spices, as well as in some medicines. It can cause rashes and aggravate asthma.

E2T 2 Potassium benzoate – as 210

E213 Calcium benzoate – as 210

E214 Ethyl p-hydroxybenzoate – banned in some countries

E215 Sodium ethyl p-hydroxybenzoate – banned in some countries

E216 Propyl p-hydroxybenzoate – a possible allergen

E217 Sodium propyl p-hydroxybenzoate – banned in some countries

E218 Methyl p-hydroxybenzoate – possible allergic reactions, mainly on the skin

E219 Sodium methyl p-hydroxybenzoate – banned in some countries

E220 Sulfur dioxide – can cause asthma attacks and metabolic changes in people with decreased kidney function also destroys vitamin B1. It is typically used in beer production, non-alcoholic drinks, dried fruits, wine, vinegar, potato products.

E221 Sodium sulphite – cleaning agent in production of juices. It is likely to cause possible intestinal disorders; see 220.

E222 Sodium hydrogen sulphite – see 220

E223 Sodium metabisulphite – treatment agent, see 220

E224 Potassium metabisulphite – see 220

E225 Potassium sulphite – see 220

E226 Calcium sulphite – to be avoided, banned in some countries

E227 Calcium hydrogen sulphite – banned in some countries

E228 Potassium hydrogen sulphite – see 220

E231 Orthophenyl phenol – may cause skin problems; can be used for agricultural purposes.

E232 Sodium orthophenyl phenol – see 231

E233 Thiabendazole – see 231

E234 Nisin – an antibiotic derived from a bacterium. It is used in the production of beer, cheese products, tomato puree.

E235 Natamycin – a mold inhibitor produced by bacteria; may cause nausea, vomiting, diarrhea and skin irritation; Typical use – in meat and cheese. E236 – formic acid – banned in some countries E237 – sodium formate – banned in some countries E238 – calcium formate – banned in some countries G E239 – hexamethylenetetramine – banned in some countries E249 – potassium nitrite – fixes color and meat preservative. May have an effect on the transfer of oxygen to the body, resulting in rapid breathing, dizziness and headache, potential carcinogen, not permitted in food for babies and children.

E250 Sodium nitrite – can cause hyperesthesia, potentially carcinogenic, banned in many countries, can interact in the stomach to form nitrosamine. It is recommended to avoid it.

E25T Sodium nitrate – see 250

E252 Potassium nitrate – see 249 and 250

E260 Acetic acid – the main component of vinegar

E261 Potassium acetate – in sauces and marinades, to be avoided by people with impaired kidney function.

E262 Sodium acetate, sodium diacetate – see 260

E263 Calcium acetate – see 260

E264 Ammonium acetate – as 263, but may cause nausea and vomiting.

E270 Lactic acid – lactic acid, acid regulator E280 – Propionic acid – used in bakery and sausage.

E297 Fumaric acid – obtained from the plant Fumaria esp. F. officianalis or in the fermentation of glucose with molds. It can serve as a flavoring agent, for acidification, antioxidant in soft drinks.

So how are you? I sincerely hope you think before you put something in your mouth. I have a habit. Before I buy something to eat, I ask myself the question:

Does that help me? Or harm? And what's more!

Smiling day, Irresistible!

You are never given a dream without also being given the power to make it true. You may have to work for it, however.

Richard Bach

Dry Heels

Have you noticed how feet only have certain places where the skin is rough? Only the heels. Only one side of the big toe. Only the smallest toe. On the side of the wide part of the foot, only on the left or only on the right. And everyone has it in different places, in combinations of only five to three points. For example, the big toe on the left, the ankle on the right and the heel.

Why is it happening?

If the body has the correct posture, the weight is evenly distributed over the entire foot, the legs are soft "like a baby's bottom." There are no rough areas. When we shift the weight of our body in a certain way, we step on specific points. If in one case 60 kg are evenly distributed at 20–25 cm in length and 5–8 cm width, the other is two or three points with a total size of 3cm. To cope with friction and pressure, the body sends stocks to make the skin thicker in the given places. Imagine the baby's delicate skin – it cannot withstand friction, right? But if we make it 10 layers thicker, it's another matter!

It is very easy. See how you have rough and thick skin where your shoes are worn.

The second reason is due to the thousands of foot creams people use. They contain many substances that suffocate the feet. It's like a plastic bag. You must have noticed how you apply the cream and things are tolerable. One night you forget it and you scrape it off the sheets.

The third reason is due to wearing shoes. If you wear tight shoes and they constantly tighten in certain places, there is friction and re-accumulation of skin.

Fourth, improper treatment. If you use curettes or rub them with a heel file, pumice and the like in every bath, you over-rub them. The body accepts it as a threat. Skin must be produced there quickly to protect the body from losing it. This is how it's taught. If you think it every day, it will produce it.

Still, everyone wants soft baby feet. But how to achieve it?

Fix your posture. Think how you walk! Think how you step! See where the shoes are worn and where the hard areas are. Think of not stepping on them.

Do not use cosmetics that are not natural, that contain harmful suffocating substances. Wear comfortable shoes. If they put you in a room just as big as you, how would you feel? Yes, the legs feel the same way!

It is easy to apply cream all your life. It's hard to get rid of the cause! Do not treat the consequence, remove the original source. The fact that the skin is rough is your least problem. This means that your posture is incorrect. And this is a far bigger problem than rough and cracked skin.

A wonderful and unforgettable day, Sweety! And don't forget to smile.

Smiling is when you look your best.

Unknown

Quick Tricks

Peeling with fruit acids
2–3 strawberries
half a kiwi
5–10 drops "Vizin" (eye drops)
Mix everything and apply on face. Stay like this for 2 to 5 minutes. Depending on how much we want to renew our skin, we can do it 1 to 3 times a week.

Lip regeneration
Mix honey and sugar
Put shea butter (maybe castor oil) on your finger and stir in the mixture. Rub on lips and stay like that for 2 to 10 minutes.

Body detoxification
Take a hot shower. Once the pores are open and the whole bath is steamed, rub with honey. Stay as long as you like. If you are in the sauna, maybe 10–15 minutes. Wash without soap.

Regenerating body scrub
Margarine (not butter) and sugar in a ratio of 50 to 50
On dry skin, rub the whole body, starting with the driest part. Then wash only with water!
Soft skin and a nice complexion:
Use cocoa butter on the beach or 2–3 times a week. It is a powerful antioxidant and regenerator. Then wash only with water!

Facial scrub
Add baking soda to your washing product. After a nice hot shower, rub the face from the chin to the forehead. The movements are from the bottom up and from the center out!

Nail whitening

Baking soda + hydrogenated peroxide + lemon juice
Spread and stand for 5 minutes.

Eye serum

Eye contour cream is placed on the bottom of an ice cube tray. Pour green tea and freeze. Rub one cube every day.

Mask for dry skin

Avocado and greasy cream (can be castor or cocoa butter). Stay 15 minutes and do it 2 times a week.

Split ends

Before the bath, apply castor oil. Not very generous! Castor oil is difficult to wash. Stay from 30 minutes to an hour and wash off.

Long lashes

Every night lubricate with castor oil.

Thick eyebrows

Every night lubricate with castor oil.

Dry lips: Never again!

Every night lubricate with castor oil.

Cracked heels

Every night lubricate with castor oil.

Dry cuticles on the nails

Every night lubricate with castor oil.

Happiness is not always doing what you want but wanting to do what you do.

Lev Tolstoy

Does a Perfect Toothpaste Exist?

Yes! You just have to know what to look for!

I am not a dentist and I will not explain to you what you need in a toothpaste to have healthy teeth. But I know what you don't need to have a healthy body!

How often do you brush your teeth daily – once, twice? And how often have you wondered what your toothpaste contains? Probably never. Otherwise, you would have stopped washing with it. We use it day after day, month after month, year after year... We spend 2,190 minutes a year brushing our teeth. Do not play Russian roulette with your health.

Let me show you why and how!

One of the ingredients used is SLS – sodium lauryl sulfate and its derivatives (ammonium lauryl sulfate, ammonium laureth sulfate, sodium laureth sulfate, TEA laureth sulfate, TEA laureth sulfate). It was invented during World War II to wash away rust and oil from tanks. Subsequently, its sparkling properties are evaluated. This is a cheap foaming agent used in over 90% of personal care products – toothpaste, cleansing gels, shampoos, masks, creams and much more. It accumulates in the eyes, liver and brain.

Next is triclosan – highly carcinogenic. The presence of the product increases the risk of heart attack and stroke.

Dyes also do not lag behind:

One of them is blue. The composition is E133 or FD&C Blue Dye No.1. Blue is not among dyes that are obtained naturally. It is most often extracted from oil. All food coloring, unless it is a pure fruit or vegetable extract, causes a risk of allergies, cancer and lack of concentration due to accumulation in the brain, heart, liver.

Cellulose gum – is not a food, it is a supplement that thickens the product. It is also found as carboxymethylcellulose, CMC or dietary fiber. It is often found in some medicines. According to research, it is not absorbed. It passes and leaves the body. However, English laboratories have shown that there is a risk of it causing allergic reactions.

Chlorhexidine – used as an antibacterial ingredient. The problem is that it destroys both positive and negative bacteria. It also kills our protective flora from internal infections. Thus, we get sick more often and have a problem not only with the oral cavity, but also with the health inside us.

Triclosan – was originally registered as a pesticide. It causes cancer, thyroid hormone disorders and affects the heart. Binds to chlorine in water.

Parabens (propylparaben, methylparaben, butylparaben, ethylparaben, phenoxyethanol) – highly toxic substances, preservatives that accumulate in the body and cause hormonal disorders.

TEA, DEA (triethanolamine, diethanolamine) – toxic, carcinogenic substances.

Propylene glycol (propylene glycol), Polyethylene glycol (polyethylene glycol or Antifreeze) – toxic, carcinogenic substances. They cause changes in the liver and damage the kidneys.

Formaldehyde and toluene – toxic, carcinogenic substances.

E210 benzoic acid – phenylcarboxylic acid. May cause asthma.

E211 sodium benzoate, E212 potassium benzoate, E213 calcium benzoate. They cause asthma.

Sorbitol E 420 – causes gastrointestinal disorders and increases the risk of diabetes.

Sodium hydroxide – has a whitening and corrosive effect.

Carbomer – is a synthetic polymer.

Sodium saccharin is a carcinogen.

Paraffin – a petroleum product, highly carcinogenic. Retains toxins and prevents the penetration of oxygen.

Glycerin – makes a film like stretch film. Protects against harmful ingredients, but also stops the useful ones that come with food.

Fluoride – when I started writing the chapter, this was the first on the list. Then I realized that I had to write an entire article just for fluoride! Otherwise, I would have lost you between the lines.

We continue with fatal cell mutations not only in our body but also in future generations – our children. If you've noticed, all the articles I write revolve around lowering metabolic age, oxygen, and free radicals. Fluoride is present in the water we drink. It's in tap water and mineral water. The amount may become too much without us noticing.

There are many harmful ingredients and there is no point in trying to remember them. If you haven't read my articles on harmful substances, read them! Search for "Toxic Beauty" and "Harmful Substances" on the site.

The problem with all of these ingredients is accumulation. They have been declared to be harmless in small quantities and the body can handle them in small amounts. But they are found in all products. A little here, a little there; finally, there is a big accumulation in our body. Brushing our teeth, applying cream in the morning and evening, our washing gel, our hand soap... we have made it a habit to use them. We are looking for something cheap. We don't look at quality. And if we see the word organic, we relax. In reality, these are the products we need to be most careful about. Don't think about how often we will eat chocolate, but think about what we brush our teeth with every day for 6 minutes. Let's look at the composition of our cream and the products we use for our daily routines.

If you do something routine, make sure it is useful for you! Let it work for you, not against you!

Smiling day, Charming beauty!
Ema

Your subconscious holds a power that can change the world. You just need to ask for it.

William James

The Long Walk

Pros and cons

The sun is shining and everyone is walking. A few days ago, the kids and I went to the sea garden. They rode scooters, and I ran. We went through the entire sea garden in Burgas – from the salt pans to the bridge and back. And I remembered a lot of things.

Those who were starting the walk had their chins up, excited that they were finally out. They walked at a faster pace, as if they were late. Those who had been walking for a long time were like caterpillars. They were walking slowly, their abdomen forward, the waist bent in a C shape, all weight hanging on the spine. Their head protruding forward. And the pelvis seemed to be waving hello. We often blame men: "Hey stop staring at her, you are married! Shame on you!" It's good that I'm a woman, otherwise I would be lynched. Have you noticed how much people flinch when they walk? No matter the gender! Or they poke out their asses as if they want their ass to say: "Look at me, look at me." They're not really to blame. It's really a muscle weakness.

I am often told: "Emche, I walked a lot yesterday, today I will take it easy." A long walk can burden us much more than a workout. It is very important how we do it! When it is warm, we melt like hell out in the sun and nevertheless, we walk. We take it slow when in fact we shouldn't be doing it at all!

Our life is a workout which does not stop! The body trains even when sleeping. Your posture in the car, in front of the TV, in your sleep, at work... it's all an endless workout. Spending 40–60 minutes in the gym in sweat and thinking why did I come is a small dot in the big circle.

How to stand better. How to be faster. How to be more precise. How to walk properly!

The walk is wonderful! You take vitamin D. You produce hormones of happiness. But when you get tired, you produce stress hormones. The body makes memories precisely when it is under stress! If there's stress, the muscles remember the way of movement and the posture, they change their habit! How do we correct spinal deformities? We cause pain to the body (spasm, tightness) until it gets tired. Why? Because when we are tired, we change the habit. Then we seal in the memory of the cell how to do it.

It's the same with walking. You are tired – the body is learning! The more tired you are, the more you remember! I love to say that the last 10 minutes of your workout is your entire workout!

Think about how you walk! Feet forward. Knees under the pelvis. Swallowed abdomen, tight lower abdominal wall waist flat. The diaphragm opens to the side to breathe. Shoulders back. Head up. Chin forward. The body should be straight like a plank. The more you get tired, the more you should think! Think how you feel!

And no! Do not wear a belt. We have already talked about how it works. Don't screw yourself up!

Move! Movement is health! Movement is life! Feel alive! Live!

Sunny day, Lovely one!

We are what we constantly do. This is why perfection is not an act but a habit.

Aristotle

On the Left ... On the Right...

At the NESEMINAR by Yuli over 250 people came to talk to me. How do I know? This is how many business cards I had with me... and they took them all. And everybody said: "I have a curvature here." Then I realized how people were focused on their pinky but not the big picture. For those who were not there, do the following thing – put your finger in front of your eyes and look at it. You only see it, right? Now focus on the background. You don't see the finger! This is how we choose to see only the problem and not the big picture.

What actually happens?

The structure of our body is very simple. Imagine many lines parallel to each other:

So, everything is fine. And this is the structure of our body, whether we look at ourselves from the front or from the side. If we tilt one of these lines to the left, the line below it and above it will shift to the right. And so, every next one will also react. We call it balance.

Thus, if we have a shift of the shoulders back like a bow, then we will have a shift of both the neck and the waist forward. If we have one shoulder dropped to the left, then our head will be slightly bent to the right and our pelvis will also be slightly to the right. If we carry the split of our hair to one side, we often keep our head up to it. If our split is on the left and our head is raised to the left. From there, the shoulders shift and we lift the right one and bend it further down until the arch of the foot falls. And vice versa. If we have a fallen arch, we can keep our head to one side. This results in asymmetry in the face. Look in the mirror. One eyebrow is always higher than the other. As a former beautician with about 10 years of experience, I would say – genetically. But I'm sure it's not! No client has two identical eyebrows. The truth is that from our way of life everyone has some asymmetry. One moment it doesn't bother us, and the next it starts with pain and health problems. Of those 250 people I mentioned at the beginning, over 90% had different phases of distortion. In other words, in some form, their spine is "S"-shaped. And those with a herniated disc spoke as if life was over and should be so until the end of their days. This is corrected with the right exercises! And relatively quickly! You can deal with the problem and straighten your spine in a month. It's up to you! Correcting your posture is not just 1 hour during training. It is thinking about the things from training and practicing them in your daily life!

So, think about how you move, how you stand, how you sleep! Make it a habit! Listen to the body, it speaks to you! The problem is, it's like a voice in the desert! It speaks a language we have forgotten. Technology is so advanced that we are waiting for everything to be ready. The boss should tell us how to do our job, they put in fuel for us at the gas station, we are given recommendations when we buy things at the store, someone teaches us how to eat. We don't recognize what we need... it's sad!

Learn to listen to it and act!

We are still masters of our fate. We are still captains of our souls.

Winston Churchill

What Is Blue Light?

Do you know that light tells your cells what to do? It programs you and unlocks various processes in you, whether you want it to or not.

Visible light has all the colors of the rainbow and starts from 380 nm (nanometer length) to 750 nm. In the last century, John Ott, a Disney photographer, discovered that different lights had a certain effect on animals and plants. For example, pumpkins placed in blue light produce only female blossoms, while those placed in pink produce only male blossoms. The pumpkin produces both blossoms and fertilizes itself. Placed under one of the upper lights it cannot do it due to its same-sex blossoming. He also found that animals placed in unnatural light could give birth to almost only males or only females, which changes when the light also changes. He also found that flowers that open their petals every morning did not do so when he photographed them with a flash several times during the night. That is, the lighting has confused their internal clock and they do not seem to get enough sleep to have the energy to open their colors in the morning.

What does this have to do with us?

We humans have two hormones that strongly affect our willingness to work and regenerate. In one case we expend energy, and in the other – we sleep at night. They are cortisol and melatonin. To put it simply – cortisol is what we want to lift and wake us up/focus. This happens artificially when we drink coffee. And of course, when the sun rises and cortisol rises to wake us up. In the morning our cortisol is at its highest, with a peak around 09:00. Then we need to be most productive if this cycle is no longer broken by factors such as the environment, food, stress, light and sleep habits. If you think you're just a "night bird" and your energy comes in the evening – my answer is no. It's just that the cycle is totally destroyed and reversed. It's as if the body only manages to wake up in the evening when it should actually fall asleep. After the morning peak cortisol gradually drops, reaching its lowest point in the evening at 18:00, which it holds until 06:00 in the morning. When cortisol drops at 18:00, melatonin rises. The job of melatonin is to calm us prepare for regeneration and lead us to a deep and restorative sleep that occurs imperceptibly. This is the optimal case and it happens very rarely nowadays.

Why?

This light, which wakes us up and keeps cortisol levels high, is blue (400–500 nm). This same light is most strongly emitted by the computer, telephone, TV, fluorescent and white LED lamps. Which means that as this light enters our eyes after 6 p.m., our body will think it is morning and will try to wake us up. Imagine falling asleep, but someone keeps slapping you... you can't sleep, can you? This is very stressful and exhausting. We will go to bed and it will take us 15 minutes to fall asleep or we will go to bed exhausted and in the morning, we will need coffee to wake up. We need this coffee because the body is exhausted from the fact that the light has lied to it all day, that it is morning – time to get up, even when it is 22:00 in the evening! Keep in mind that in order to sleep well, get rested and be energetic and not hate every morning, we need to have low cortisol and high melatonin before bed.

How to achieve this?

I will add that our body has evolved on this planet with the cycles of the sun and moon. And it continues to check with them, not with our desire to stay up late. This means that from 10 p.m. to 2 a.m. it recovers physically, and from 2 a.m. to 6 a.m. – psychologically, regardless of whether we went to bed or not! The difference is that if we do not lie down, this recovery is simply insignificant!

Melatonin, in turn, is produced from 9 p.m. to 1 a.m.

Therefore, sleep between 9 p.m. and 1 a.m. is the most effective and indispensable. If you are not in bed between 10 p.m. and 2 a.m., your tissues and organs cannot recover. For people who work night shifts, it is almost impossible for me to lower their metabolic age. I've been struggling with this for 6 months now and I'm failing! This only proves to me the fact of how important regeneration is in these hours.

If we go to bed after 10 p.m. and if we sit in blue light in the evening, it is equivalent to eating sweets all day – we raise blood sugar, gain weight and are tired, we want sweets or coffee. This happens during the day. But in the evening it is even stronger.

How do you lower cortisol and raise melatonin in the evening for optimal sleep and even faster sleep? After 6 p.m. we need to block as much blue light as possible (400–500 nm) that enters our eyes. The simplest way to do this is to put programs on the phone and computer that block blue light. For phones there is a program called Iris. It is a world-famous Bulgarian program that has a simple free and optimal, as well as paid version. And the second is twilight. Launched on the phone along with the free Iris, it brings an acceptable amount of red, which neutralizes the blue. Iphone has this option from settings – Accessibility, and computers can download f.lux and adjust to 1200K, which is quite good. Screens turn red because red is the antidote to blue, raises melatonin, calms us and reduces eye strain. Oh yes, blue light from the screens is what leads to myopia, pain and tension in the eyes and even inflammation throughout the body, which I will explain another time. If we like the above programs, we can take a step forward by ordering glasses that completely block blue light and put them on at 6 p.m. in the evening (like UVEX for $ 9 from Amazon). This will prepare us for bed in time and we will feel much more rested the next morning. I used to go to bed at 11 p.m. and midnight and it took me 8 hours of sleep to sleep well and a few minutes to fall asleep. Then I used the aforementioned programs, but still each bulb had a blue light from which you cannot escape. When I started wearing glasses blocking blue light at 6 p.m. and red glasses at 8 p.m., I started going to bed before 10 p.m. and I could sleep well not for 8 hours but started waking up rested in 7 hours! I have clients who without using any glasses, just by using those programs and going to bed at 9–10 p.m. instead of 1–2 a.m. started sleeping enough for 7 hours instead of 11!

This helps us gain not only energy but also time! Time, multiplied by the energy you have, determines how long you can live and what you will achieve in your life.

What happens if we have too much blue light during the day? We become hyperactive, irritable and gain weight.

We have evolved on this planet with sunlight. Sunlight has almost as much red light as blue. During the day, the two balance. When our computer or lamp is a lot bluer, it's like putting an alien sun in the sky – our body gets confused and overwhelmed. It tries to activate too much, which exhausts it. Example – when my computer lights up normally, if I stay for 5 hours, I fall asleep and I am exhausted. If I block enough blue light from it, I can sit all day and not feel tired from it.

Okay – what are the best lamps for the day? They should be as yellow as possible, but even the yellowest LED lamps (2700K) still have too much blue, and the fluorescent lamps flash constantly and lead to bloodshot eyes, headaches and other problems. Old normal incandescent bulbs that are not energy efficient have the closest blue-red balance to sunlight and are best for our physiology.

Studies show that even a directed point of light behind the knee raises cortisol, so in the evening we should sleep in a completely dark room, without lights from routers and flashing phones, with thick curtains. The clock in our head needs 30 to 90 seconds of light in the morning to know that the sun has risen and to begin the processes of waking up, raising cortisol and lowering melatonin. So, in the evening, if we get up, we need to be in a very dim light, because by turning on the lamps interrupts our regeneration, whether or not we fall asleep again. Remember what it's like not to sleep all night and let the sun rise. We feel real fatigue when the light comes in the morning. Our body wants to rest, but the sunlight entering the eyes tells it it's time to wake up. It's like we are "dying to sleep" with someone on the other side pushing us all the time and telling us "get up, get up, get up!"

Sunlight also has ultraviolet light, which has been shown to be useful to us and is blocked by any glass window. Therefore, when we can, we stand at an open window during the day and in daylight. When we can't, it's nice to add ultraviolet light bulbs to others which will feel like you are letting the sun into the room. Also, red LED bulbs can balance white light from others. A red light in the evening 1–2 hours before bedtime leads to the deepest regeneration you will feel.

Tendons

As a hard gum or elastic
Why do we train and what role do tendons play? For every 10 people, 9 have stretched some part of their body. Over 50% of injuries are in the tendons, not the muscle. **Why?**

What does a tendon actually do? It attaches a muscle to the bone. When the muscle tightens, it pulls on the tendon and it moves the bone. That's how we move.

When I was little and we were preparing for the next competition, I had to learn to do twine in one day! Because the girl who performed it got injured. I did it! And I tore a tendon. The problem was not that I did it in one day, but in the way I was taught to do it. Springing!

Some time ago, every coach, when he had to stretch you, adjusted you, stood behind you or in front of you and pushed or pulled. I sit on the ground, spread my legs apart, someone sits across from me, fixes my knees and pulls me towards him. Or he stands behind me and pushes me to the ground. In both cases we spring. What is happening? The muscle stretches, pulls the tendon. It starts to hurt – this is a factor that the muscle contracts back. And at this point we press again. It is the muscle that is in spasm, contracted and small, and we are stretching it with force!

If we want to stretch properly, we fix until it hurts but acceptably. And we hold for 30 seconds. Then lightly press 1–2 millimeters more. And again, we hold. Then another 1–2 millimeters and again. And so, 3 times. Gradually the muscle and tendon relax.

Separately, we need a massage in areas where we have overstretched muscles. And not a massage with a masseur. A **self-massage** – a lot of pain in a short time.

I will not do it alone, so I announce the time and date and I know that on this day I will relax with 12 other people. This is a painful thing, so that if you are alone, you will give up. We hunch because one muscle is tense and the other is weak. We have wrinkles, often from overexertion, not from age. We need to find where the adhesions and pain are and eliminate them.

Let's go back. At school, you sit at a desk and run your hand under it to pick up a textbook. But instead of it, you come across old gum. One that dried a month or two ago. This is what your tendons look like! Rigid tendons equate to a high risk of injury. If we fall from a ski, a bike or just slippery ice, either we break a bone because we are heavy and have worn calcium in the bones over the years, or the tendon is hard and torn. It cannot respond to muscle pulling.

Second option – you reach for the textbook and under it there is gum stuck from the previous class! You pull and it stretches. You can't remove it from the textbook. Oh, no! What happens to this type of tendon? Doctors call them "loose joints." The inability to pull the tendon from a muscle in a given direction. It stretches in excess. If we stand all day in a hunched position that pulls the joint on one side only, we stretch the tendon on one side only. Thus, one side is as tight as the old gum and the other is as loose as the new one.

Your tendons are important! Do not ignore them.

If you ignore them – you ignore yourself!

Dandruff and Hair Mask for Straight Hair

From my 10 years of experience and my work with clients, I realized one thing: food, cosmetics and stress – these are the culprits for dandruff, skin eczema, dermatitis, seborrhea and scalp flaking.

Why?

1. Food – fast carbohydrates and sugars feed candida. If without them we have a simple reddening of the scalp, after beer, chocolate and the like it begins to flake and grow.
2. Stress – if we have constant stress, lack of sleep, if we are even just 2 minutes late, there is enough stress for the body not to have time to regenerate. The immune system collapses.
3. Cosmetics – look at the composition of your shampoo, conditioner, stylists and everything you spray and apply. We take in more substances through the skin and hair than through the mouth. Are you sure what you put in it is okay?

We have already passed the harmful substances. If you skipped them, go back and take a closer look. If you don't take care of yourself, there is no one else to do it!

So, look at what you have in the products and don't read the big label! Nor the Bulgarian label! Read the small print on the back!

On the Internet you can find everything on this topic.

Everything you read here is based on my experience. And the experience of the people I helped. As well as based on research that was given to me as an example when I was studying.

When I started practicing in the field of beauty, my first teacher had a degree in veterinary medicine. But she was a teacher of cosmetics. And she told me the following: "If you have irritation of scalp or fungi on the feet and hands, buy antimycotic spray from the vet pharmacy. But take the transparent one, not the yellow one, it costs about 18 leva." The idea is as follows. No one has time to treat their animal every 14 days or do 20 treatments, if not for life. Everything in veterinary medicine is concentrated. While our products are made to be used for life. They suppress. You use it – no problem. You stop... it's there again. This is a trick I pass on from her to my clients. And over 5,000 people have tried it in the last 10 years. Everyone already has this spray in the fridge. Me too.

In one article I promised you a mask for shiny and straight hair. And now I will share it with you. Are you ready? Make your favorite tea, nice aromatic coffee or the drink you love the most. Make your own mask! Feel the rich aroma of chocolate! Sit down for 30 minutes, open your favorite book and give yourself a moment just for yourself! Feel how your senses are nourished by the scent itself. Feel how your emotions change! Enjoy!

For shiny and straight hair at home mix:

2–3 tbsp. chocolate (I use cosmetic chocolate. It costs 15 leva per 1 kg and is suitable for firming and anti-aging masks for face, body and hair. It is not edible.)

1 tbsp. Castor oil

1 banana – without the peel!

You can add egg yolk and any other oil you have on hand. Including cocoa, coconut, butter, grease – the ones we eat and have in the fridge. Here it is very important to puree it!!!! It needs to have a creamy consistency! Otherwise, you risk brushing your hair for 2 hours in the bathroom due to the pieces of banana stuck to each hair!

Be thankful for what you have and you will have more of it. If you concentrate on what you don't have, you will never have enough.

Oprah Winfrey

SOS!!! Hair Loss!!! SOS!!!

Plus Bonus Recipe of Magical Hair Mask

These days I am all about the hair, so I will share something more on this topic. Spring and autumn are seasons in which they always make us drink vitamins, tablets and powders. Our immunity is dropping. We may feel exhausted and without energy. But hair loss is a must. The hair is dry at the ends, greasy at the root. We take a bath and "SOS, is there any hair left on my head at all?" Entire locks fall out!

Correct. Something is wrong. But what?

1. **We lack minerals**

    Here we must check what kind of salt we eat (remember the differences in salt?). It's in the beginning!

    How much water do you drink? – If it is above 0.033l per kilogram you dilute them. If you drink coffee, green tea, etc., dehydrating, add 0.500l. And we commented on free radicals and water as well!

2. **Dehydration** – we do not drink water in the cold. And we should. Then the hair loses shine and elasticity!

3. **You use hair products with harmful ingredients**. Recall the article about harmful substances in cosmetics. When you have any of these substances in your products, they make something like a stretch film on each hair. Thus, they create a greenhouse effect and dry the hair until it becomes like straw and pulls every drop of life out of it. Not to mention how it affects the scalp.

4. **You wash your hair too often** – the more often you wash and treat it, the more it dries and breaks. The hair is washed every 3–4 days. This is the normal cycle! If you want to wash it more often – something is wrong.

Remember the oily skin of the face and over-washing? Well, it's the same. The more you dry it out, the faster it wants to produce sebum. At one point, instead of greasing for 5 days and producing 5 tablespoons of sebum, it learns to produce it in 24–48 hours. Many clients have told me, "I must wash it every day, otherwise I don't feel good." Start stretching the washing time, and in two or three weeks you'll see how things work out.

5. **You walk without a hat** – Have you watched *Tinkerbell and the Secret of the Wings*? What happened to the wings of the fairy in the cold? They broke! In the cold, hair is like a small fragile strand. It freezes and breaks. The sharp temperature difference inside to outside is even worse!

6. **Food** – if you eat sweets, it breaks down collagen fibers.

Hair loss. Imagine the trees in the fall. What is happening? The leaves fall to protect the tree and keep it alive. In winter it cannot feed them. They freeze from the cold. So is the hair. It sacrifices itself so we can survive. To sacrifice oneself for the good of another does not sound to me like "everything is okay. Keep going!"

For me, hair loss is the red light: something is wrong. Check what!

I know I confused you a little. The last page and a half had many reminders of things already said. The goal was to put the whole picture together for you. I used to give you pieces of the puzzle, but now you see what it really is. From all the training I do, I realized that you can't understand the end if we don't start from the beginning. That's why I don't have short lectures. All my events are all day or 8 days. Either you will learn and understand everything, or it doesn't make sense.

And now I will share with you how I fixed my hair loss after giving birth. How I made it grow like a weed! And how today

I do not bother to cut it, because it does not get split ends and does not stop growing!

For long hair without hair loss mix

1 tsp. honey

1 tsp. alcohol

1 tbsp. fat

1 tsp. almond oil

1 tsp. Ikarov hair mixture (it contains a lot of oils so that you don't have to buy one by one)

1 tsp. glycerin

1 tsp. castor oil

1 tsp. Trivitaminol (purchased from a veterinary pharmacy – Vit. A, E, D)

1 egg yolk

It is very important to do this for no more than 3 months and to rest for at least 3 months. Observe the expiration date of Trivitaminol and keep it in the refrigerator! Leave on the hair from 30 minutes to 1 hour! Not more. Otherwise, we will have an allergy because the ingredients are very strong.

Swelling of Legs, Fingers, and Entire Body
Lymph issues!

Be not another, if you can be yourself.

Paracelsus

Why and how to fix it?
Let's start with Why?

1. **Weak muscles!** If the muscles are weak, they do not have the strength to push out the fluids that pass through them. Lymph and blood are stagnant! The blood should carry a glass of smoothie filled to the brim with an umbrella and a straw every 4 hours. In fact, it carries it every 6–8 hours, without an umbrella, and it spilled half on the way. The cells are hungry and not functioning properly. The lymph, in turn, must pass to collect the empty cups and straws, clean where it has been spilled, take the pots and throw them in the cauldron (kidneys). Yes, but it doesn't work. It is slow and instead of cleansing every 4 hours, with the congestions it reaches for 6–8. Do you remember what happens when the garbage truck doesn't pass? What if it's 48 hours? And two days? Month? Year?

2. **Distortions** – any distortion is like a dam for a raging river (blood and lymph). We have talked many times about how distortions affect our body functions. And I also mentioned to you the 6-week free "Let's Stand Upright Together" campaign at home, which you can take advantage of.

3. **Chronic diseases and postoperative edema!** I have worked with a lot of people. I will never forget a Russian astronaut, he was 43 years old, retired. For three years in a row, he took a course of 10 pressure therapy procedures

with me every summer. He told me how three times a year it was a must for him because his lymph was not circulating due to the lack of gravity in space. We have treated many swellings after operations to remove the ovaries or lymph ducts due to cancer. When you close the highway, the small roads become congested. From gravity everything falls down, but does not return. In the beginning, swelling begins, the legs are soft and just like a shaking mass, resembling jelly. At this point, movement and creams that enhance lymphatic circulation help. If we do not take measures, the legs increase in volume to 3–4 times. They become heavy. If we press them, our fingers leave light marks like pits each time for a long time with white dots. From the fluid, the lymph becomes a jelly that thickens and thickens. The incoming lymph no longer passes, the legs become cold and very hard. They are no longer just slightly sensitive, but completely lose their sense of touch. There is also salvation at this time. Heating products, combined with draining. The best I have worked with are the Spanish brand "Tegor" and specifically their professional drainage series (oil, serum, mask, cream). But this was 2012–2015. They are found only in salons or directly from their representatives in Sofia and Plovdiv. The best results are when mixing electrical stimulation – it trains the muscles and makes the muscles move, liquefy the lymph, and then use the products and do pressure therapy. It is very important how the pressure therapy is done! It is not done the same way each time. It starts very lightly and intensifies every time. There is no way to take everything out from the first time. If you try, you will have varicose veins. When I received this treatment, it was in such a way that after 5 sessions I had varicose veins on my left leg. Then, I learned how to apply the treatment and it was something else. We should not feel pulsations as if our heart is in our legs and we feel it beating. You can't use straw to make a waterfall! **Everything is gradual!**

4. **Pregnancy** – during pregnancy the body begins to store. This is genetic. But we can minimize it with proper diet and exercise.

5. **We ate** white salt, sugar, white flour, gluten or dairy products! If you enter our site semma.bg, I have made four pictures in the free category. I have shown clearly which product causes what on the face. This way you will understand what does not affect you well and what does not harm you. In this case, the main problem with it is the toxicity, fluid retention and the processes they cause. In the morning we are swollen, rings do not move, the legs are swollen as if we have not slept. We need a ton of makeup and skinny jeans that we can barely get into to hide the damage. The body has the ability to retain 1 to 5 kg of fluid for 24 hours.

How to prevent swelling?

1. Be careful what you eat by avoiding white salt, sugar, white flour, gluten and dairy products! Or at least what affects us! How to find out – by reading the articles about these products. Each one has precise signs which make it recognizable. All of them will be in my new book.

    (Here I will give you a joker: If you take a picture with my book and send me the photo to my personal e-mail emiliq.belcheva@semma.bg I will give you a 15% discount on my new books, video trainings, video lectures or from a personal consultation. Just choose! Enter semma.bg/zateb and I have another surprise for you.)

2. Do we exercise regularly. If after sports we are swollen, this means we don't do it right.

Right means with the law of biomechanics used in corrective gymnastics.
3. We sleep in the right position!
4. We think about how we move – we must be upright!

It's not hard! You just have to want it!

You will never be too old to set a new goal or dream of something new.

Clive Staples Lewis

Flat or Fluffy Belly – Who Is to Blame?

Cortisol and other suspects.

I don't know anyone who doesn't want a six pack! And I know few who really succeed in a healthy way. The market is flooded with magic pills and appliances, but how many of them work in our favor? In our minds, the equivalent of a flat stomach is hunger, deprivation, stress. It's terrible!!!

Weight gain in a certain area is due to a certain hormone. People often tell me: "I only gain on my ass!", "I only gain on my stomach!" This is because each hormone affects a specific area. Remember the lights on the dashboard of the car? Well, belly equals high cortisol levels. Do you remember blue light?

What is cortisol? **This is the stress hormone.** We synthesize it under stress, lack of sleep, starvation.

When we have high levels of cortisol, we

increase the loss of muscle mass,

slow down the metabolism,

reduce fat burning,

gain fat in the abdominal area,

maintain low testosterone levels (strong fatigue, less strength, etc.),

damage tissues and organs,

the regeneration of the organism is slowed down,

we feel constant and easy irritability,

we feel constant fatigue for no apparent reason,

we are weepy,

we have accelerated pulse, and

we have high blood pressure.

I think it's enough.

In order to have a very toned abdomen, women must have 10–11% body fat distributed throughout the body. Less than 10%, periods disappear and hormonal imbalance is 100%

"upside down." In order to have a nice shaped belly, we must have 12–15% fat. Men in turn must have 10–12 %. How does this happen? Definitely not with starvation.

What does stress mean for the body? "Something that disrupts its normal function." Hmmm let's see:

1. Insomnia – our body should sleep 6–8 hours. From 9 p.m. until 1 a.m. we produce melatonin, from 10 p.m. to 2 a.m. we regenerate physically, from 2 to 6 a.m. – mentally. When do you go to bed?

2. Improper training – you train only for the abdomen. You only stress the abdominal area. The body does not lose weight in one place. It loses weight completely! You kill yourself in training and for two days your body hurts badly. This is stress. It's like someone beating you up and then wanting you to smile. Hard, huh?

3. Food – eating too much fatty, processed and canned foods directly prevents weight loss, no matter what and how much exercise you do. This prevents the reduction of fat on the waist and abdomen.

   Most diets say: do not eat greasy! Healthy fats, monounsaturated and polyunsaturated fatty acids help reduce body fat. They contribute to the proper division of cells, the regulation of metabolism and the melting of adipose tissue around the waist. We don't accumulate fat from fat! We have already talked about how food affects emotions. Improper diet equals depression, stress.

   Lack of fiber – fiber contributes to the burning of belly fat. Fiber regulates metabolism, blood sugar, insulin, gastrointestinal function and weight. Fiber releases toxins and creates a feeling of long-lasting satiety.

   I am regularly told: "I do not eat salt!" And why??!?

   There are over 72 microelements in salt that you need!!! With them you build tissues and organs. Imagine a white sheet, glue and a colored sheet. If you have all three, you can create everything. Now imagine you don't have glue! You put colored pieces onto the white sheet, you create a miracle, but you lift it up and... everything is on the ground. Everything is unstable, fragile and impermanent.

Eat salt! but eat large, gray, greasy sea salt unrefined!

Alcohol, white flour, white sugar, refined salt equal 100% stress. They cause infections in the body. We have already talked about sugar and salt.

4. Lack of magnesium – with magnesium deficiency we have higher levels of blood sugar and insulin. This causes an accumulation of belly fat. Consumption of foods rich in magnesium lowers blood sugar and insulin, accelerates fat burning and reduces the risk of diabetes. Foods rich in magnesium are avocados, dark green leafy vegetables, nuts, seeds, fish, legumes and more.

5. We eat fast – our stomach is full about 10 minutes before our brain tells us. Today we are distorted from our daily lives to eat very fast. We eat for 10 minutes. That is why we often feel our stomach is heavy. The role of the teeth is to tear the food prior to swallowing. First, we eat 2 times more, second – in large pieces! How to digest and assimilate food like this? We are still swollen and heavy.

6. Skeletal and muscular dysfunctions. Atrophy or overexertion in muscles cause bends, distortions, congestion, lack of nutrients.

7. We have fungal or bacterial infections. A month ago, by coincidence, I ate outside. The next day my stomach swelled with whatever I ate. I gave a test sample and had streptococci all over my body. Bacteria do not stand still. My skin became rough. My face wrinkled. My heels were scraping on the sheets. My pores widened. I got acne and I haven't had it in years! I was hungry nonstop...

I cured myself. But I am unlikely to eat outside again in the next 6–9 months. Many people do not feel that they have something because they do not know what it can be and what it causes. And again, they cause a lot of stress to themselves.

The body is not stupid!

Belly fat is the most dangerous excess fat in the whole body. It endangers health and life. Excessive accumulation of fat around the abdomen and waist increases the risk of diabetes, cardiovascular disease, cancer and hormonal problems.

A tight stomach means, above all, a healthy core! It means that you have the right posture, you breathe well, you eat well, you have good lymphatic and blood circulation. The metabolism is at the correct level, oxygen flow is great, the regeneration of tissues and organs is 100%. So don't say, "It's genetic!" Think about which of the things listed above you are not doing and what you are doing!

I wish you an unforgettable day filled with many smiles! Because you are beautiful and you deserve it!

I didn't have work days or off days. I just did something and I enjoyed it.

Thomas Edison

What about you?

What Is Cellulite?

What is cellulite? At first glance, the nightmare of every woman, no matter thin or overweight. This is a stagnant and storage phenomenon in adipose tissue, namely a violation of the microcirculation of the blood and lymph. Do you remember the theory about the river, the end of which is at its beginning and the thousands of dams?

Each person has a subcutaneous fat layer, which consists of many small bubbles separated by connective tissue. In women, estrogen is responsible for the structure of these fibers and their location perpendicular to the skin. Normal skin (without visible traces of cellulite) is characterized by the presence of many small fat cells, grouped in fat sacs.

What are fat cells? This is a reserve in the body, which is formed by sugar and its derivatives, white flour, white salt, pasteurized products and the wrong combination in food.

These foods cause inflammatory processes in the muscles. In order not to get sick, the body consumes part and the other, encapsulating it in fat bubbles and storing it for processing later. The problem is that "later" never comes because we are constantly taking the next dose. Separately, the inflammatory process releases cortisol and insulin from the rise in blood sugar and panic in the body. When we have insulin (lowering blood sugar) or cortisol (stress hormone), the body only stores, not uses. We feel overwhelmed, it's hard for us, we don't have energy and we want 7 to 1 to remove the unnecessary ones. It's genetic. Centuries ago there were no clothes and heating, no air conditioners and refrigerators. Women had to gain a lot of weight in the fall to be able to feed their babies and themselves, give birth and recover without food. Unfortunately, the body remembers and this dependency is still valid. The problem with us is that these kilos are not lost after the winter but become more every year.

The aforementioned foods make us addicted to them. When consumed, they increase fat cells, and they release the hormone of happiness, endorphin. Everyone wants to be happy. When the blood sugar rises, insulin is released, it lowers the sugar lower than necessary, the energy drops. Cortisol is released from stress, we start to gain weight, we start to get depressed, feel whiney and need constant hugs. And we eat again. And again, and again, and again... If we get used to eating more than we use, then our fat bubbles start to grow and swell. The connective tissue between the fat deposits, which attaches them to the skin, pulls the skin down due to gravity, and the fat layer pulls up. Many swollen bubbles on the buttocks and thighs appear.

The men did well. Their fat layer penetrates a wide network of longitudinal and transverse fibers, which tightly hold the adipose tissue and allows even an overweight man to look tight. Complete injustice! Due to all the hormones and especially estrogen, which we take with milk, chicken and food, this is already beginning to be observed in men.

How is cellulite formed?

Due to the structure of connective tissue, cellulite is inherent in every woman, regardless of weight.

In nature, nothing is accidental. If we press on the skin and orange peel skin appears from one place to another, we are ready to accumulate fat reserves for a possible pregnancy. This is the first stage. We lie down, everything is smooth and beautiful, but if we get up, the whole truth shines. The skin sags slightly and there are bumps in places. At this stage, the normal circulation of blood and lymph is disturbed, the tissue acquires a swollen appearance, although still in a minor form.

The second stage. The effect of "orange peel skin" is noticeable when both lying and standing. Swollen fat cells are grouped into fat nods, causing tissue fibrosis. As the nods grow, as well as their thickening and hardening, the skin surface becomes uneven. Thanks to the circulatory disorder, the buttocks become cold to the touch!

How to decrease cellulite?

Food

Get sugar, white flour, pasteurized dairy and white salt out of your diet! As I mentioned, fat cells secrete endorphin which reaches the brain and gives us a sense of satisfaction. Just as the squirrel collects acorns for the winter and is happy to see her barn full, so she pulls the sweet and the harmful. The more fat bubbles we have on our butts, the more we want to eat sweets. This is how the dependence is formulated, which we can get rid of only by limiting these products.

Exercise and going to the gym improve blood circulation in problem areas and burn fat deposits to make energy. Here it is very important not to lose weight fast. Rapid weight loss means weakening the organism! There are many harmful substances in the fat deposits, closed like in a cell dungeon. If we release them, we can quickly get poisoned. On the other hand, the skin does not shrink for a day.

Massage

Self-massage improves blood and lymph circulation in problem areas. The purpose of the massage is, in addition to circulation, to break down fat deposits and to remove through the lymph the products released from the oxidation of fats, and, also, to help restore the skin.

Massage is effective only with proper nutrition and exercise. When fat cells do not grow, but shrink, and when we waste more energy than we take in with food, then we improve the metabolism and blood and lymph circulation in the problem areas.

If you want success, you should look successful already.

Thomas Moore

Types of Cellulite

In the textbooks you can find 6 types of cellulite, and in different textbooks the types are named differently.

After 10 years of practice, for me, cellulite is mainly divided into two types: hard and swelled.

What is swelled or soft cellulite?

There is hard cellulite under the surface, but there is a lot of retained fluid on top. The texture is soft and shakes when walking. If we shake our legs or buttocks, they continue to move even after that. Here we must stop consuming white sea salt, Himalayan and salty foods (not salted by us). Let's start consuming only coarse oily gray sea salt. Let's stop drinking colossal amounts of water and wash the necessary microelements from the body (we already talked about how much water we need to drink). Let's start eating every four hours. Here are suitable drainage procedures and sports that have a drainage effect. If we do everything correctly, then in 2–3 weeks all the hard cellulite will come to the surface and from a soft consistency it will become rough with visible cellulite. And so, phase 1 is over.

What is hard cellulite?

First case:

It is most common in athletes and people who train incorrectly. At this point, the energy from the food is more than the energy expended. No destructive procedures are applied, only force. The muscle grows around the fat deposits and although the leg is very tight when pressed or when the muscle is tightened, small dips are visible (orange peel skin).

Second case:

Anyone who manages to get rid of swollen cellulite or does not retain fluids has hard cellulite. These are fat deposits that have accumulated over the years, have strong joints and have become solid. Do you remember the chewing gum under the desk? The longer they stay under the desk , the harder they become and the harder they are to clean.

In these cases, we need a change of diet, procedures to break it and sport that breaks it, thermal products with which to lubricate the skin during training to enhance breaking. They do not need to be expensive, but we need to feel warm, there is hyperemia (redness of the skin). Of these, it is very important not to smear where we have varicose veins, on the face and around the heart. Everything else is "welcome." Here we are not looking for quality, but only the thermal effect.

Do things with people who you share common goals with.

Warren Buffett

Anti-Cellulite Procedures and Recipes for Anti-Cellulite Scrub

How do we know if what we are doing is working now and not after 10 procedures?

For 10 years I have been dealing with anti-cellulite procedures, sports, cosmetics and diets in order to eliminate cellulite for clients! I have worked with over 8,000 people with this focus, we have lost thousands of kilograms and we have tightened meters and meters of skin! And let's get to the question – how do we know if this works for us?

There are two types of procedures – breaking and drainage (cleaning).

The first type are all manual massages, vacuum massages (with suction cups or devices), there is vacuum in combination with infrared light, LPG, and in Russia for two years, a very popular device based on vibrations, which stimulates the muscles and breaks them at the same time, cavitation and much more. Here the goal is to break down fat deposits.

Who needs this procedure? Anyone who has visible dips (orange peel skin), as well as hard cellulite.

How do we know if it works? To undertake such a procedure, the small dips between the fat deposits must be visible. After the procedure, if the work is done well, the treated area is soft, fluffy and shakes like jelly. To the touch, we feel how the consistency of the surface is soft and smooth.

The second type are drainage procedures. These are all cardio workouts plus manual or hardware lymphatic drainage. Until two years ago, only one lady in Stara Zagora performed medical manual lymphatic drainage in Bulgaria. It is very specific and special tightening bandages are applied. Choose only medical devices. One such is BTL, called pressure therapy. What is it doing? It works like a blood pressure monitor. Applying pressure to the legs, it compresses the legs, squeezing out the retained and unnecessary fluid (lymph and blood). Until now, on request, medical devices have blue legs. There are many Korean ones on the market, costing 1,000 leva each, with orange legs that tighten only to the thighs, leaving all the fluid in the buttocks and causing varicose veins. There should be no pain or pulsations during the procedure. If there are any, then at this point in this place the fluid that wants to pass is greater than the capacity of the blood vessel and the procedure can cause varicose veins. There are specific ways of using the device and each time you have to apply it harder than the previous time. If the pressure is the same every time, do not pump more than the previous time.

When should it be done? After a breaking procedure. Drainage is performed when we have swollen feet, when the consistency of cellulite is soft and shaky like jelly. Then the solid deposits are too deep and there is no point in a breakdown procedure. You can only use cosmetic creams to enhance the effect. It is good to wear leggings on top of the cream. So we put on cream, put on special leggings, which on one side is nylon, on the other – fabric and enter the machine. There is good hygiene and there is no danger of transmission of fungus on the feet and other infections.

Recommendation: before the first procedure, as well as on every third one, do a peeling. Otherwise, the creams and dead skin create a barrier like stretch film and do not allow the new dose to penetrate deeply and work.

Shared knowledge is valuable knowledge. Share and let it be useful for as many ladies as possible!

Recipe for homemade anti-cellulite scrub!

4 tablespoons freshly ground coffee

4 tablespoons ground coarse sea salt (looks greasy, gray and dirty)

1 tablespoon coconut oil

1 tablespoon grape seed oil

Mix everything (if necessary, more oil can be added). Then add the essential oils:

10 drops of orange

5 drops of lemon

5 drops of lavender

You can replace the oils as follows: rosemary, lemongrass, grapefruit, geranium, juniper, ivy, dill, oregano, cinnamon, cloves – each works differently and depending on the type of cellulite you can make the best combination for you!

Massage the problem areas with this scrub 2–3 times a week for 5 minutes. It is recommended immediately after playing sports. Why? Do you remember the types of anti-cellulite procedures? This scrub causes drainage. Very soon you will notice how the skin tightens, has elasticity and density, and cellulite is reduced!

The two most important days of my life were the day I was born and the day I found out why.

Mark Twain

I Can't Come, I'm on My Period!

"I need to stay close to the fridge"!!!

Whether as an excuse or as a reason we believe in, this is a commonly used phrase in our head.

What is happening?

Let's look at the big picture: Depending on the point of view, ladies' hormones fluctuate. Why?! Men are always on the same hormones, mainly affected by stress and food. Women change every day. We don't have 3 identical days a month! Our hormones range from complete happiness to total depression, from anabolic effect (muscle growth) to catabolic (breakdown). But here comes the good news! We can easily lose and gain weight if we know when and how to!!!

Let's look at the average 28-day cycle. It goes through 4 phases. Progesterone and estrogen range from low to high. When we have estrogen (from the seventh to the fourteenth day) we grow. When we have progesterone (from the fourteenth to the twenty-eighth day), we break down. The problem is that when we have progesterone, the levels of serotonin (the hormone of happiness) are lowered. The body temperature rises, the blood thins, the blood vessels constrict so that there is no great blood loss through the uterus. The cells are hungry. There is a shortage of substances reaching them. It's like drinking diluted coffee through a crushed straw. Not only do you barely drink, but it has no taste!

We are starving!!!!

A large amount of cortisol – the stress hormone – is produced.

Panic on the max!

We only eat sweets. By eating white sugar and white flour, we cause infections in the body and more stress. Separately, with a large intake of carbohydrates, blood sugar rises, which releases insulin, which lowers it back. To make matters worse, it does not lower it to the norms, but below them. After 30 minutes we are hungry again and again, and again, and again...! Finally, our period ends, and we have gained 3–4 kilograms! The problem is that before menstruation we need more calories – about 100–200 per day. But from the wrong diet and the amount of sweets, we take much more. During menstruation, we no longer need these calories on top. Not only do we continue with 200 unnecessary calories more, but we also eat another 1000 extra ones!!!

Second bad news: Women are more prone to knee injuries than men and according to statistics from 2017 this risk is 3 to 6 times higher on a certain 10 days of the month!

Why do we swell? To dilute the blood and let it pass through the narrowed blood vessels, in order not to become dehydrated during blood loss. And because we ate Himalayan or crushed white salt. (We discussed this in detail in the article on salt.)

Menstruation: In these 3–7 days our circulatory system is greatly increased. The uterus and ovaries apply pressure and raise the internal pressure in the abdominal area. If we have a weak lower abdominal wall, we feel swollen, as if we have swallowed a basketball. If we have weak muscles in the vaginal area, when lifting weights, we have the feeling that something is pushing us strongly down from the inside. This sensation may be a slight pressure but can lead to severe pain.

How to help ourselves!?!

- Fatigue and exhaustion – move! Your body is a battery! The more you use it, the more it produces! Eat animal fats, not sweets. If you want to have batteries like Duracell, eat boiled eggs with soft yolks, eat fatty meats, eat bacon in an omelet or otherwise. You need good cholesterol to make hormones. Imagine you have 10 units of cholesterol, 4 of them will be for progesterone, 3 for cortisol – so far stress hormones. Two to three for melanin or other living – supportive and what's left? 0! How can you produce the hormone of happiness or any other necessary when you have nothing? It's like wanting your car to run without fuel.

- The body begins to retain water – eat only coarse sea salt, gray and greasy at first glance. You lose blood, you lose minerals! In order to restore the quality of the blood, you need to consume minerals.
- It's harder to concentrate – don't eat fast carbs that raise your blood sugar too much.
- Add turkey, soybeans, legumes, pumpkin seeds. These are foods rich in the amino acid needed to produce serotonin – tryptophan. Separately, soy is known for its content of female hormones that will help you in difficult days. There's a catch here. Do not get used to it because it's totally genetically modified!
- Train with light weights on difficult days, increase rest time. If you feel discomfort, see where it is. This is a weakness. Remove it! Work on the lower abdominal wall and that doesn't just mean abdominal presses! Tighten the uterus, tighten the vaginal muscles! Learn to breathe! Train for a diaphragm! Improve blood oxygen saturation. Your workout strengthens your blood circulation, so you will nourish your muscles. Yes, the bleeding is slightly increased – watch for it! Learn to feel your body. If you have pain in the ovaries (as I did) it is quite possible to have shortening and tightening of the muscles next to them. If you massage and relax it, you will not have pain during the period.

Be strong enough to know you can't do everything by yourself.
Unknown

Blackheads

Today, everyone is horrified to look in the mirror and see a bunch of blackheads. We use all sorts of masks – some tighten, others dry out and peel off, others sting... We enter the bathroom and look forward to steaming and then squeezing each pore. And then we put on a kilo of foundation to mask the effects. And so, every month.

Have you ever wondered why they appear? Why does the skin get oily?

One of the reasons is milk. All dairy products cause blackheads. This is because of pasteurization, which is required if purchased from the store. Also, from casein inside the milk. In the human body, the casein: albumin ratio is 1: 1. In all other milks casein: albumin is 3: 1.

It's like drinking a triple shot cup of coffee. That's why babies have colic if Mom eats dairy. But that's another topic.

Dairy products make the chin thicker, more sensitive and slightly rougher. The forehead is full of light, tiny pimples with white tips. Or it may just appear uneven.

The second reason is cosmetics. If we have harmful substances, they make a film like stretch film. The skin above it is beautiful. Below it is moist and acidic. Fungi and bacteria develop. It's like putting a plastic bag on your head and breathing in it. Oxygen is running out. And all the skin becomes condensed. The pores open, moisture comes out and the skin becomes dehydrated. To compensate for the oil, we apply drying and anti-acne creams.

It is much easier to use natural fruits and vegetables (as in the article on fruit peels) to renew our skin. Blackheads disappear on their own when we fix our diet. Chips, semi-finished products, smoked meats, dairy... they overwhelm us.

Instead of squeezing every month and hurting your skin, do an exfoliation! After a bath on nicely steamed skin mix soda with something. It can be with your washing gel, maybe just with a little water. And get a massage. From the chin to the forehead, from the center to the sides.

For a few days smear on your face something that you eat. Cucumber, strawberries, melon, banana, watermelon... Give air to your skin. Once you feel like eating, you need it. When you have a need, you are in deficit. And until it reaches the skin, you have to fill the deficit.

And the next time before you get angry at the blackheads, think about what your body wants to tell you! Something is wrong! Do not mask it with makeup. Don't hurt yourself every month. I clean my face once a year! But before I got to that point, I cleaned my food. When I was a beautician, I cleaned it twice a month! There is a difference, isn't there?

It's like saying black is white. The truth sooner or later comes to light. **Don't mask it but be the first to figure it out!**

A magical day, Irresistible!

Fluoride (F) – For and Against

After the toothpaste article, I couldn't hold it any longer. You need to know this too!!!!

In Charles Woody's book *The Fluoride Deception*, according to Dr. Phyllis Moulenix, former director of the Forsyth Dental Center in Boston, USA, fluorides are highly toxic to the central nervous system and can have a detrimental effect on the brain, even in low doses. In infants and children, brain development is impaired, motor function is affected, and the ability to learn is reduced.

Even 20–30 mg of fluoride a day disrupts calcium metabolism and as a result the bones become brittle and fragile.

The main way to fluorinate is through aluminum. Remember the caramel cream bowls, the soft ones. And all the aluminum dishes? It is a very dangerous metal and accumulates directly in food. Therefore, if you have such vessels and you love each other, get rid of them now!

Let me give you more examples of why:

In 2012 Dr. Mihail Todorov commented on the latest research in the United States as follows:

> More and more scientists are claiming that one of the biggest deceptions of humanity is fluoridation – toothpaste, water saturated with fluoride. We think that we enrich tooth enamel with fluoride, that we keep our teeth healthy and beautiful. But the situation is the opposite – it is a fraud.
>
> Concerns have long concluded that the best way to get rid of harmful industrial production is to sell it to people who will use this crap. One of the most dangerous

global crimes of this kind is the fluoridation of water and toothpaste.

Toxic fluorides began to accumulate in large quantities during the production of atomic bombs in the United States as part of the Manhattan Project. The vegetation died, as did all the domestic animals in the area, and residents filed lawsuits against Dupont,[sic] then hired lawyers and doctors to find a "healing application" for fluoride. The result was the false theory sucked out of their fingers that fluoride strengthens teeth. The DuPont concern came out of the lawsuit dry and was given the perfect opportunity to dispose of the toxic waste by selling it to Americans for domestic consumption.

In the 1980s, fluoride was found to stimulate bone growth. But unevenly, causing bone deformities and mutations. In 1988 in the United States, it was declared a strong carcinogen. Turns cells into cancer.

Shortly afterwards, Procter & Gambel published a study that "Fluoride in drinking water causes genetic damage. In human tissues, fluoride causes chromosomal aberrations, which in the United States alone kills 50,000 people a year. In addition, the link between fluoride and premature aging of the body, the destruction of collagen, i.e., connective tissue, the immune system, genetics, etc. has been proven. "

In 1990, fluoride was shown to affect the pineal gland. It is located between the two cerebral hemispheres. It regulates the release of melatonin – a hormone that helps regulate sexual maturity and protects the body from the harmful effects that free radicals have on the brain.

Dr. Jennifer Luke of the University of Surrey in England proves that the pineal gland is the first to fall under the blows of fluoride. According to this research, the excess of fluoride in the pineal gland leads to serious dysfunctions, provokes early puberty and reduces the body's ability to fight free radicals. According to this study, fluoride can provoke a genetic change in the fetus during pregnancy and increase the risk of cancer. Many studies show that fluoride can cause bone cancer.

At the energy level, the pineal gland is responsible for the body's adaptation to new vibrational parameters of the earth.

Fluoride is known for its false protection against tooth decay. But the problem is that it is in food, whereby flouride accumulates in the body.

Uncontrolled use of fluoride is dangerous to health. It destroys catalysis – a group of enzymes that protect the body from the harmful effects of free radicals. Remember the article on free radicals? They destroy cells, threaten the integrity of DNA and cause mutations in cell reproduction. The chain reaction of cellular mutations can cause the formation of cancerous tumors.

Recent research in the book *The Fluoride Deception* by Charles Woody has shown that there is a link between Down Syndrome and water fluoridation. Pregnant women are most at risk because excess fluoride in drinking water enters the mother's blood and hence the fetus' blood.

Fluoride is found not only in toothpastes and cosmetics! It is found in drinking water, in tap water, in our eating and cooking utensils. In mineral waters it varies from 0.3 to 5. Therefore, I will repeat again: read the labels!

I advise you:

1. Do not use aluminum containers.
2. Do not use tap water – for cooking and drinking.
3. Do not drink drinks from metal cans. And read the labels. Must be explicitly written "does not contain fluoride."
4. Do not consume anything from canned metal.
5. Pregnant women should not drink tap water.

6. Do not water the fruits and vegetables you grow with tap water, as it contains sodium fluoride which accumulates in the soil and passes into fruits and vegetables.

    Think, Beautiful! Think and take care of yourself!

    Because you are the only one in this world who can help you!

    Ema

Tighten, Get Slimmer, Stand Straight!?!

Summer is coming and more and more people ask me how they can lose weight. And then, "But I don't want to stand upright, I want to lift my ass because it's shapeless. I want to tighten up a bit! I don't want to lose weight. I want to look good!" etc. Then: "I am cleansing. I eat only fruits and vegetables, no meat. And I do a lot of exercise" (they haven't exercised so far because it's been winter). And so on.

If you're reading this, you may have asked me some of the questions. The above has been gathered from about 30 consultations in the last 2 weeks. But it all revolves around the same thing. Now we will remove one of the SEMMA groups (7.30–8.30 p.m.) and replace it with a group for corrective gymnastics. You'll find out why in a moment.

Let's start one by one
It all starts with straightening. And straight to the example – Me! For 4 years I trained for over 6 hours a day. I was in the gym, I ran 15–20 km every day, I trained for 2 hours of gymnastics, more than an hour of break and what not. I was perfect! With clothes! Without clothes, my legs had a lot of cellulite. And only a slim woman can understand that. I was also teaching spinning. As a coach I had a bunch of workouts! The cellulite was still there. My food was the same as it had been for the last 10 years.

The difference? For the last 2 years I have been doing corrective gymnastics on a spinning bike. I don't have a gram of cellulite! Even when I press my thighs together. I stood straight! Do you remember the article about the river? How everything in us is like a river? Lymph and blood are one big river. The end is at the beginning. Where you bend, it becomes a dam! What's going on around the dam? We are gaining! The tissue does not feed, does not clean. Cellulite is a blockage. Cellulite is storage. Cellulite is an atrophy of the tissue caused by compression and poor circulation. Obese people come and tell me, "I don't feel it." Fat compresses nerve endings, touch receptors, heat receptors, cold receptors... They don't work.

Everything goes hand in hand! There is no way to be hunched over and without cellulite. There is no way to be hunched over and not have retention of waste (fluids, lymph, toxins, fat).

Diet? I wrote a whole article about "Nutritional plan VS Diet" on the site. Before that we talked about "Metabolic type" and what it defines. There I described in detail what happens after a diet and why we gain weight. Why we feel deprived. And how, if we eat right, we will not feel deprived because we have no desire for sweets, sugar, white flour. We don't think about food for at least 4 hours. Not for a coffee, not for a candy... nothing!

Why do I say no to detoxification with fruit and vegetables? Because they don't have value! Everything alive on the planet is made up of protein. It is plant and animal! Many people say they will detoxify themselves. They start eating only salads – lettuce, parsley, onions, tomatoes, cucumbers, red beets, carrots. So far, no protein! The body begins to have a deficiency and inability to absorb trace elements. We start adding cheese and olives. Remember the article about salt? You like yellow cheese, for a while – the perfect ratio between protein and fat. It is genetically encoded in your brain. But today there is no fat or protein... everything is pasteurized. It interferes with the function of your hormones and disturbs the balance in the body. Fruits – sugars, glucose, fructose. The article about sugar? It's great! Read it if you missed it. We start wanting dates and dried fruits. This is due to lack of energy. Energy comes from animal fat and pure glucose. The difference is that glucose is like a dose of fast fuel. And the fat is the stove that works all night. You choose whether you will be on doses or on solid fuel! Being balanced or up and down... that's the question!

You do the cleansing. You eat your own muscle. If you are a vegetarian and you know well which vegetables have protein and everything you need – okay. But those who ask me are not! The body panics and enters a mode of accumulation. You have no energy. If you combine it with training, it becomes a peak and you lose weight. Shock dose... as they say. You're eating yourself! You are satisfied. You stop! You start eating meat and everything again. You reduce your training because the vacation is over. And you gain not 5 kg (which you lost), but 10. And it's just summer! Great!

I have many clients outside Bulgaria who practice Reiki. In order to pass certain levels, they are forced to cleanse without any meat. Why? The meat is acidic. All dead food – cooked, boiled, baked, heat-treated – is acidic. Remember the articles "Alkalinity VS Acidity," "Cancer" and "Free Radicals"? Yes, that's the point. You reduce dead food, you increase living food. You become alkaline! You become charged! Your energy goes up. But we don't feel the technology around us that dulls our senses. We've lost our senses little by little from the food that kills us! There are practices that try to enhance it. The issue is they know nothing about food and anatomy! For generations people kept saying to exclude meat, but why has been forgotten. We have eaten a lot of fresh food in the past. By "fresh" I mean picked just this moment, not standing in the store or driven from the other side of the world. Picked green and ripened in the truck. The negative charge is alive for about 48 hours. Everything alive is negatively charged. It charges us! Neutralizes free radicals.

Relax! Every problem has two sides. Many people throw themselves headlong into training. You are overweight, have cellulite, hunching, pain... because one muscle has atrophied and another has overstretched. There is no way to tighten the loose if you do not loosen the tight. It is no coincidence that once a month I do a full body self-massage. And it's no coincidence that I'm making a group about it. First – when I have a group, I am serious! Otherwise, I will think of dishes, laundry, this, that... And I will give up. The idea is once a month for 3 hours – you relax the face, head, neck (remove wrinkles), arms, shoulders, chest, abdomen, back, legs, buttocks, fingers... everything!!!

Conclusion!

Stand upright! Learn to breathe! Turn your routine actions: how you sit, sleep, eat, drive the car, walk... into training! They regularly tell me: "I don't have time!" You move all day! Life is training! The meaning of training is to become better at what you do outside the gym! Not to break yourself in 40 minutes and recover in 2 days! After training you need to have energy! Open the diaphragm. Breathe! Hold your chin up. Feed your brain! Take away the swelling! Be productive! Enjoy! Remove the dams! Clean up!!! Release the emotions! Leave the suitcases with negativity behind you! Smile!

The body is a machine! The perfect machine! We are born perfect! We break down along the way, not by age!

Stop thinking about which diet to do. Do something for yourself in the long run! Stand up! Everything else happens by itself!

Smile, Beautiful! You are most beautiful when you wear only your smile! Ask your husband.

Nothing really stops you. Nothing really bothers you. Because your own will is in your hands. Remember your character is your fate.

Unknown

Say Yes!

In the last year, I learned something that works a lot. I decided to share it with you! Our beauty depends on our inner state. And that comes from our mental beliefs and convictions. Today I will not talk to you about masks, substances, food or training. I'll tell you a little secret that I already know works.

Collect the "yes" in your favor. Have you noticed how in big seminars, in books and even in my articles we constantly ask you questions? The purpose of these questions is to turn off your brain, more precisely its negativity. If you once said to yourself that the sea is green, no matter how much I argue with you that it is blue, it will be a lost cause. The brain does not like to make mistakes. What normal person likes to lose!?! But this often plays a bad joke on us.

If you're reading a book to develop yourself, to change, and you don't agree with the author, if you're in a lecture and you're just wondering when it's going to end, and a bunch of things like that, you're not going to get anything. You will waste your time and be disappointed! Your brain will not remember even 1% of what is said or read.

However, if you agree with what is written, it remembers. This is a very easy trick. It doesn't matter if you are reading a recipe or a complex project. If you say "yes" three times in your mind, you will remember everything after that. Yes, but on three different facts. The sea is pink – yes, mermaids swim in it – yes, and the foam is vanilla – yes! From now on everything else will be recorded as a recorder in your head! But you have to say it!

I love reading and learning new things! Some rest with a movie, others when they go to a disco, and I rest with a good science book!

I used to read something 20 times to remember it. Now I say "yes" out loud three times for the first two pages and from there the book is sealed in my head. I may not know which book I learned from, but it is a fact that I learned it!

So, collect your yes. Find something to agree on! Make your development easier and faster!

Save time! Steal your most valuable and non-renewable resource – time!

Say yes to yourself!

Sunny day, Fairy!

Either I will find a way, or dig it.

Unknown

How to Kill Bacteria Plus a Russian Recipe that Is Ages Old

I decided to share with you a Russian recipe that has been passed down through the generations of a family of healers. To understand how much power there is in it, I will only insert two introductory sentences. From the creation of Russia to the present day, there are only four famous Russian healers. They were called "Kalduns." In the history of Russia, only 4 prizes "Contribution to Russia" have been awarded. I am fortunate to know personally the son of one who received a prize and the grandson of the other who followed in their footsteps. The recipe was given to me by Sergei (I will spare his last name, due to his request), the grandson of one of the Kalduns.

How do I know it works?

I had to try it with my family. At the request of my daughters, I enrolled them in kindergarten in the same group. And yes, you will say here, but they are 2 and 4. And yes, they were in the same group. Due to the breakdown of the diet and the intake of huge amounts of carbohydrates only, the internal environment of their bodies turned from alkaline to acidic. So, they became susceptible to bacteria. You will say that this is normal. Yes but no. Most of the healthy children in the kindergarten are carbohydrate metabolic types. And the fact that there is a lack of protein does not interfere with the functioning of tissues and organs. Mine are not! Once the body is acidic, it is an ideal place for bacteria. They caught streptococcus pneumoniae, haemophilus influenzae, moraxella catarrhalis. For 7 months they took antibiotics for 6 or 7 times and the only thing that happened was that a fungus appeared – Candida albicans. They were good for a couple of days... and again. In the third month they were admitted to hospital. Iva had pus in both ears. The doctor who operated on her urgently said that in another 15 minutes she would have ruptured her eardrums. Not to mention the danger of meningitis. She was on intravenous antibiotics. I will not comment on how the problem was not found after three times in the emergency, going to the GP and homeopath. She couldn't hear for the 5 days we were in the hospital and I had the feeling that my hair turned white. And again, the bacterium survived!

She was discharged. No more kindergarten! We changed her diet and things were okay, but the bacteria were there. One candy, a little more carbohydrate and everything was on fire again. After the seventh antibiotic I decided it was better to live with the bacteria and without sweets than antibiotics. Each antibiotic was prescribed after examination and antibiogram. I found everything I came across for the given bacteria. I have experience working with the treatment of fungi such as Candida albicans and different types of bacteria. I had made long lists of herbs that affect them. From there I remembered the recipe that Sergei had given me two years ago when we worked together. I found the main herbs to which almost all bacteria are sensitive, added them to the recipe and the result was obvious after 3 days, after the seventh day we gave a sample for an antibiogram that came out clean!!! I'm not saying that it will help everyone, because people are different, but it helped a lot, and we were one of them.

The magic is as follows:
Make tea by boiling 500 ml of water and add:

- an equal teaspoon of coarse sea salt (we have already talked about how to choose one with minerals)
- 5–6 grains of cloves
- cinnamon stick
- 2 cloves of garlic

- 2 stalks of thyme
- 1 pinch of oregano
- walnut (preferably with the shell, if not – only walnuts)

If there are a lot of secretions, you can add a packet of black tea and just a pinch of baking soda.

We drip one dropper in the morning, noon and evening. If it's for a child, always try it on yourself. If you overdo it with salt and soda, you can burn the mucous membrane of the nose. It doesn't sting, if there is a sting it is local in a particular place, not in the whole nose. Do not make the child lift his head up too much, because in very young children, if there is a lot of snot, instead of the liquid going to the throat, it will go to the ears.

The tea is ready for use in the next 2–3 days. Then a new one is made! An indication not to use it is a sour smell.

Simultaneously with the drops, drink tea prepared as follows:

- boil 1 liter of water
- put thyme – 1,2 pinches
- oregano – the smaller the child, the less. The maximum is one pinch, to 3–4 small stalks
- cinnamon stick
- 5–6 cloves

Boil for 3 minutes, simmer for 5 minutes. An adult drinks 1 liter per day, a child – 500 ml. They begin to strongly nourish mucus from the lungs. If the cough is very strong, oregano should be reduced.

Oregano is not used as a tea every day, unless there is a problem we want to cure. The treatment is 5–10 days. If the expectoration decreases, so does the oregano. Until we completely remove it. The above described oregano tea can be drunk every day during flu periods and there is no risk of illness. If one day you don't have time to make tea, just put a cinnamon stick and cloves in your big water bottle. The more concentrated it is, the stronger it is.

For the last month I have shared it with over 25 mothers who have positive answers about the action. I will be happy for anyone who was helped by the recipe to write a comment on our page and share experiences. Let's not use loads of drugs when we can cure ourselves with only tea from 6 ingredients.

Why Does Hair on Eyebrows and Eyelashes Fall Out?

Have you noticed how there are months when you don't use an eyebrow pencil or shadows to emphasize your eyebrows? But there are also months when there are very small holes in your eyebrows. Why?

Sugar may be responsible for this. It causes the breakdown of collagen bonds. Thus, the quality and quantity of collagen in our body is reduced. You remember the article about collagen.

Stress – stress means production of cortisol! It affects many functions in the body. When cortisol is present, the body is in the process of gaining weight. Imagine in the fall how leaves drop so that the tree does not have to feed them. They sacrifice themselves for the good of the whole system.

Eczema or local dermatitis – we have already covered this in the article on hair loss. Disease causing chronic redness, itching and discomfort. Here comes the intervention of a doctor.

Improper hair removal – no matter how the hair is removed, it is important for us to be careful. The eyes often lie and if we shape our eyebrows ourselves, one has a high risk of being different from the other. Not to mention that every 9 out of 10 has an asymmetry and the eyebrows are different in general. You should also keep in mind that hair can only grow back a "limited" number of times before it disappears forever. Therefore, if you exceed it by plucking your eyebrows, you may eventually lose it.

Medications – some drugs cause hair growth, others hair loss. So read the leaflets.

Metabolism – metabolic disorders lead to growth retardation. In this way, the lashes fall out, but the new follicle does not develop fast enough to replace it. So, we lose more hair than we can create.

The solution

Reduce consumed sugars and their derivatives (glucose, syrups, etc.).

Increase daily intake of folic acid, minerals such as sulfur and silicon, vitamins A, B3 and E.

For eyebrows, smear with rosemary oil and castor oil, you can also add almond.

For eyelashes, massage them with olive oil or castor oil before going to bed.

After cleansing makeup, boil 100 ml of water and pour 1 packet of chamomile tea (or 20 g of dried herb). After 15 minutes, remove the packet, soak a cotton swab and make a compress on the lashes for 2 to 5 minutes.

Both eyebrows and eyelashes can be treated with castor oil. It stimulates the growth of new hair, so be careful where you apply it. Moisten a cotton swab with a few drops of castor oil and apply it every night by gently tapping around the lashes. Or lightly put it on your finger and smear.

After 14 days the results are visible: Are these your lashes?

Fruit Peelings

Today, the industry spews creams, peels, masks, serums and what not to renew, exfoliate and regenerate the skin with cucumber, milk yeast, proteins and acids, vitamin C and the like for whitening. Why? Because there is someone to buy them!

For 10 years I have tried many products and brands! I have always worked with very expensive ones! Sometimes just one product from a brand is good quality; buying every product from the brand is not worth it. There is one product that is good and the rest are being sold because of it. I mixed 10 brands in one procedure. Here it was very important to know how the pH changes after each product. This is the only way we can connect them! It is a fact that cheap serum for 9 leva for 100 ml, to cream for 600 leva worked together to give maximum results. A result that expensive cosmetics only did not give! And the finale – I always had something natural added by me! Be it a mixture of herbs made as tea and frozen in doses for lifting or bleaching purposes, or a mixture of freshly squeezed fruit juices. Be it snail caviar, frozen and clean. There was always something natural! Otherwise, the effect was 70%.

That's why customers appreciated me! I did not follow the protocol! I studied each product separately!

Why am I telling you this? To understand that the most expensive products are not always good! And that cheap isn't always bad! That often what is in our fridge is worth it!

And now I will give you a trick! A secret that I have been studying for 10 years!

Every year there is a time when the skin is weaker. More tired. You noticed, didn't you? A time when you can't go out without foundation, mascara or eyeliner. Well, it's time to update!

Start buying fruit! Start eating fruit! Do not overdo the fresh juices. I already told you – they are 50% fructose. No fiber, and you are causing internal fat – the cause of 30–40 years of heart attack, stroke and the like.

Smear the face with fruit every day. It has fruit acid that will not hurt you! You leave it on from 20 minutes to an hour. You can apply it once, when it dries again, then again. And so, from 1 to 3 times. Massage yourself with the fruit, not just smear it. Use strawberry, citrus, tomato, apple, banana, pear, grape... Whatever your soul wants. If you feel like eating, you need it. If you need it, your skin will be happy too!

Then wash only with water! And put on cream. I recommend doing it in the evening, so as not to wash your face and dry it. In the morning you wash only with water. If it is oily, use warm water, and to shrink the pores and refresh it, use lukewarm or cold water!

And think! Feel it! See how your skin feels after each fruit! If you pay attention every time, your brain will start to notice it. And most importantly – remember it! And next time it will tell you, "Hey, smear yourself with strawberries! No, no, this time use a banana. I want something more saturated! Then, I want a watermelon! I want freshness!" You will see how your skin will be different in 14 days!

Don't wait to grow old and lose your radiance! Do it when you want. Once a week. Once a month. Give yourself this pleasure!

Yogurt and cucumber, in addition to renewing and whitening. Try it! **Be different!**

If you like it, share it. Let's help the maximum number of people in the world to live happily! To live healthy!

I wish you the freshest day! Filled with smiles and positive emotions! You deserve it!

Only one person can make you happy and change your life. You.

Unknown

Cleanse!

Spring and autumn are suitable for cleansing and change! And do you know why? Why are there actually fasts? Why eat only certain foods?

It's fun! But it is forgotten!

And it took me a long time to figure it out. It took me 4 different methodologies and many years of work to see it through. And I will be happy to share it with you!

In winter we eat only dead food! This is baked, cooked, boiled... heat-treated. It is a positive charge. Do you remember free radicals? These may shorten our lives. They make us old. It depends on them how we are inside and out. Live food is now cut off, fresh. It is negatively charged! It charges us! Everything alive has a negative charge. We have -70.

Winter depletes our reserves of negative charge. In a few months we are saturated with pluses and we no longer have minuses to neutralize them. We feel tired. Sluggish. The skin is yellow, grayish, greenish. We lack brilliance.

In summer, the body gets used to the good. With the onset of autumn, we start cooking and baking again. The body reacts with fatigue. But gets used to it. It begins to use its supplies and spends in the winter. And so, we turn. From summer to summer. I know you've noticed summer rejuvenates you. The skin glows, cellulite is treated, you feel alive and energetic. You get hooked. It's no coincidence that most babies are made in the spring!

Fasting means to cleanse and alkalize the body. Remember Alkalinity versus Acidity? Yes, that's the whole point.

And here I will insert something else.

Many of my clients and friends are involved in spiritual development. Vankata and Hrisi – yoga, Ivelina – draws mandalas,

Galya and Adi – reiki... I can go on a lot, but it doesn't make sense. The idea is that any such teaching requires purification before you begin.

The meaning of purification is in the strengthening of our negative charge. More negative charge, more connection to the universe! A deeper connection with ourselves! You've heard of energies, haven't you? I know you are energy! Everything in the universe is energy. Whatever your energy is, you attract it!

If you are sick and weak, you attract it! If you are healthy, radiant, happy – that's what you attract!

Strengthen yourself so that you can give to others. This is the idea in the teachings. What do the monks do? They stand by themselves! What do they eat? Clean food! How many cases have you heard of escaping to the mountains and being miraculously healed!

Our body is a machine! A machine that can be regenerated! The point is to let it! It regenerates physically from 10 p.m. to 2 a.m. and mentally from 2 to 6 a.m. For this purpose, it needs a negative charge, micro and macro elements, protein and others. You need to turn on the regeneration light. Regeneration is unlocked by a red light (sunset). This is encoded in you and there is no escape.

And before you jump to the next fasting, think! Before they make you not eat meat and other products, think! Think what the point is!

To saturate with a negative charge! It is only in living products! And if you are going to cut out some things, do it right! Do it with sense! You don't have to eat dead food to recharge! But to eat more live food than dead! Because even if you are the best reiki master your energy runs out! And the worst thing is that you take someone else's! And if you don't learn to turn it into a negative, you shorten your life to help someone else!

Did you see yourself in any line above? I am personally in every single word in my articles! That's why I write them so personally!

Sunny day, Wonderful!

Everything you need to do to be sexier is smile from time to time.

Peter Andre

Different Points of View

Today I will not speak to you about sports, food, when to go to bed and how it affects your health. A lot has happened to me in the last week and my brain has switched to an emotional wave. For 10 years I have been dealing with emotional intelligence, management and personal development for myself. And today I decided to share with you a piece of my knowledge.

I have a strange habit: I wash the dishes every night and turn off for 20–30 minutes. This is my way of analyzing what happened during the day. I speak aloud and it's just me and the sound of running water. Everything else doesn't matter. This is how I learn from my mistakes, analyze what and how it happened. What caused it and whether it is a consequence or a reason for something else. Pluses and minuses. At this moment it is 28 May 2018, 10:19 p.m., I listen to Vivaldi's "Four Seasons" and I let my mind pour out on the blank sheet.

There are two ways of accepting the world!

One is to allow what is happening to you to crush you. And the other is to charge you and make you give even more of yourself. You can see every mistake in people and allow them to irritate you or like them as they are, knowing that they give their best and you just demand too much!

When I listen to music, I only hear motivation! I hear them sing that my dreams are in front of me, how I need to move forward, how no one can stop me, how everything is in my hands. How did this happen? Listen to the music! There are two types of songs. Some motivate you through pain. They sing about how you are hurt, how vulnerable you are, how the world ends... and the only way to avoid it is to take matters into your own hands. The other type is motivation through success. They sing to you of how the dream is in front of you, how much you can achieve as long as you ask for it! If you're like me and you're motivated by opportunities, you don't have to listen to the first kind of music. It will crush you!!! It will chew you up and spit you out without blinking and you will feel constantly stagnant. I solved this problem by changing the station every time there was no motivating music. You'll be amazed at how many things this trick can accomplish.

If someone told me a year ago that I could work for pleasure, not for money, I would laugh at him! Today, 7 months after I decided to drop everything and do only what I like, I do 5 workouts a week instead of 12. I work with only 18 people in training. I lead for pleasure. And I earn enough through individual consultations and trainings. I used to wonder how to fill my gym, now it is my vacation!!! And the feeling is unique!!! The people I pedal with are friends with whom, instead of poisoning our lives with cigarettes and coffee, we gather to pedal and prolong our lives!

Why am I sharing it with you? Because in the last month, I've heard 1,000,000 excuses around me. And not only from you! And no, I will not order people! On the contrary, I want to share something with you. I know you read my articles and this is especially for you!!! For those who have shared personal things with me in the last month.

When we want a change, the brain automatically refuses it. It finds a million excuses for not doing it. This is the only way it is calm and secure. It is afraid of change. When we have a personal consultation and you tell me a bunch of reasons "why," when you are my friend and you write to me: "I want to be like you, you succeed, and I whine all night because of...", when you tell me: "I am such" or you give me reasons why to do something... you do not convince me. You convince only yourself! And it does not matter what I tell you! You have already made the decision!

I trained so many staff in 10 years. I trained beauticians, salesmen, masseurs, manicurists, coaches, receptionists and what not. At first, I was angry that everyone was starting a job, giving them know-how and disappearing after a few months. Everyone asked me: "Why don't you sign a contract for two years, that's how you will keep them." How do you keep someone who doesn't want to stay? At first, I was angry. Very angry!!!

While after 5–6 years I realized one thing: everyone left because they had the motivation to be more! Many came with the words, "I have the experience, but I don't have the confidence to open a salon." And a few months later, they opened their own salons. They wanted employees to become employee managers. To me it is unique to make somebody be more than they wanted!

For me, there is nothing accidental in this world. **Everything happens for a reason!**

And let me give you an example. Me!

I opened a SPA center in Burgas. I was called to Sveti Vlas 3 years in a row. I rejected the call. My landlord raised my rent knowing that we invested 80,000 leva in the Turkish bath, thinking we wouldn't move out. Well, we did move out. I went to Vlas. I had employees. There was no work! Zero! My beautician left me, I had to fill in because I couldn't find anybody else. Anti-cellulite procedures were the same. But I filled in there too. For 10 days my schedule got full for the next 10 days. I was working from 9 in the morning till midnight in two offices at the same time. I invited a 62-year-old lady to be my assistant, my cousin Rumi and she was doing a great job!!!

For 3 months everybody knew about me. And thanks to my Russian clients my level reached the sky. I was near actresses, plastic and vessel surgeons and what not. On the third year the person who invited me there, Petar, sent me an SMS "I leased out your space, please vacate." And it was 20 days before the season was starting. I told my clients I gave up because I had no work. I offered my manicurist to pay a symbolic rent so she could stay, and she accepted. I rented a place on the next street, but they told me this cannot be a parlor. Well, I made it into a gym. For a few days I found a space 100 meters away from the previous parlor. It was the right choice. If it wasn't for that I wouldn't meet the lady who got me interested in face building. I wouldn't be able to adjust the knowledge I had in my head like today. And now I wouldn't be working all over the world but staying at a seasonal position in the two offices and be happy waiting for the next season. I will now skip about 10 of the same stories.

We can either get depressed and waste time in self-pity, or we can accept that it is for our good and wait for the outcome. Until then, let's do our best!

We do not need to convince others that we are right! Every time you try to convince someone, you try to convince yourself! And the biggest mistake is to get angry that the other person doesn't accept it! In fact, you do not accept it!

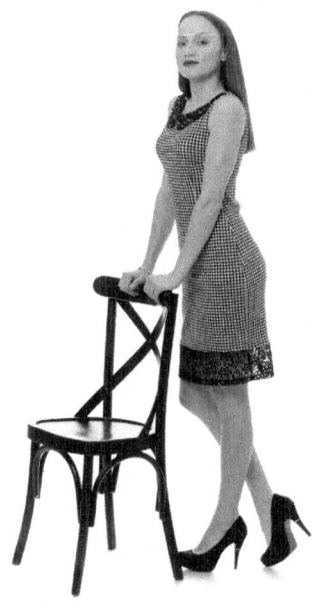

Today I was faced with a dilemma. To be angry because a very close acquaintance of mine, who changed me and helped me grow, decided to be selfish and pursue his dream, abandoning mine or supporting him! And do you know, I decided to support him! Because maybe he's done his part in my life. And you need to help someone else. And I need to pass the ball on. You remember those little tricks, how someone does good and like a ping pong ball this goes on.

Yes, I admit, first I got angry and then I ate a whole cake. Accordingly, I felt sick and barely had a workout... But I am emotional by nature. And it took me 5 hours to make sense of it.

Before you decide to sink into black thoughts, think not "Why me?", But "What's next?" See the positive side. Stop wasting time, because this is the only resource that has no return! Unless you have come to lower your metabolic age.

This is just a joke.

Well, it is too long but I think you get my point. Find your way of motivation and make it a lifestyle!

Smiling day, Fairy!

World awaits your enchantment.

Every obstacle gives a new opportunity. Every obstacle is a test.

If you smile while no one is around, then you make it real.

Andy Rooney

Trick the System

Have you ever considered that you program your brain by yourself?

If not, then in the following lines you will understand how! It is basically unconscious until you realize that it can work in your favor.

An example of this is advertising. They program us every day. For example, we associate Coca-Cola with happiness, family, satisfaction. Apple – with innovation, authority, class, quality.

Do you remember the experiment with Pavlov's dog? You click the lamp, you feed once, twice, three times. Finally, you click the lamp, the dog is drowning in saliva, and there is no food.

This is what happens with coffee, with cigarettes, with sweets, with white flour, with going to the toilet. Did I confuse you? Let me show you.

Cigarette equals a minute for yourself! A moment of calm! Cigar equals solving a big problem that we need to consider. Alcohol equals we want to turn off, to forget, to relax. The blood vessels first tighten, then open, and we get a false but satisfying feeling of freedom. This is how we really age our circulatory system. White flour and sugar equal creating a new fat cell, releasing the happiness hormone endorphin. Cake equals birthday, shared moments with loved ones. Feeling happy emotions and satisfying our need for attention.

But everything so far is false! We accept social norms and emotions without thinking about whether it is real or not. Then we wonder why our society has gone in one direction and everyone is the same. Don't you want to be different?

When I go to the playground with my kids and someone offers them candy, and we say we don't eat that, they look at me like a mother Cerberus. I deprive my children of the joy of life. I teach them from an early age that we don't have to have a birthday to get a cake. And if one day they ask, we buy it. Or we make it. For her birthday, Liya wanted to make her own cake from bananas, nuts and honey. And Iva asked for strawberries, raspberries, bananas and kiwis. And they made it all by themselves!

The brain learns. And if you teach it that your reward is something that makes you healthier, it will want that. If you are told that your reward is chocolate, it will want chocolate. I regularly hear threats like "If you don't do this, I won't buy you chocolate." At one point, the brain accepts that chocolate is the reward. And the lack of it is the punishment.

This is the trick in diets as well. The forbidden fruit is the sweetest. We start gaining weight from the lack of it, just from the thought that we can't eat it.

I changed my habits at the age of 24. Totally! I didn't want my children to feel deprived. And I changed myself. The prize is strawberries, raspberries, homemade yogurt, fish, nuts... and so we have fun every day. If we feel like eating something sweet, we take it. But it's ice cream, several times in the summer. Candy or cake, for no reason. And that's 10 times a year. And we eat them with pleasure, not with a guilty conscience that we have eaten rubbish again.

Change your attitude and you will change the habit. This is how you change your perceptions and above all yourself!

You are the one who tells the brain what it needs, which helps it; which brings it pleasure.

And if a two-year-old can do it, what are you waiting for? Find out why you want it. What are you hiding, what are you looking for? What is the emotion you crave? What is the emotion you need? And get it.

That's not how you help yourself! You just procrastinate.

Nobody cares what you hide in yourself. No one can make you feel an emotion unless you consciously ask for it.

Come to your senses!

You are Magical! Just look at where you hid your magic!

I have time and I will wait for you. The question is – how much time do you have?

They say motivation doesn't go on for long. Well, freshness after a bath too. This is why they are worth taking care of on a daily basis.

Zig Ziglar

Happiness is nothing more than good health and bad memory.

Albert Schweizer

Gluten Mania – Part 2

We've already talked about what gluten is. Since this is a really serious health issue, I will give you some more ready-made information. Let everyone think about what he eats and what he gives to his children.

Let's start!

I explained the basis of gluten, its composition and how exactly it "sticks" in our body. I also shared with you a list of foods that contain gluten. Below, I will reassure you that life without these foods continues. Even more fascinating.

The reason at the bottom is that gluten is broken down slowly... really slowly. As a result, digestion also becomes slow. I remind you that the digestive system comes first when you want to see a beautiful workout result. There is no way to have a healthy body outside with clogging inside. Fact!

Gluten is added to improve the taste of food. With this, however, the risk of gluten oversaturation loses control. I said it once, I repeat again – read the label!

Due to this fascination of manufacturers today, gluten intolerance is one of the most common allergies. In addition to food allergies, there are two other types of indigestion – food sensitivity and food intolerance. The difference is in the strength of the body's response. The body's response to this "irritant" is expressed in the construction of antibodies and substances. Yes, but they sometimes cause inflammation. The body can react in hours, it can take days.

In short, gluten breaks down the small hairs that make up the absorbent part (ganglia) of the small intestine. When they are gone, the inner wall of the intestinal tract becomes smooth. The surface of the small intestine is reduced. So, we need more time to absorb. But because our intestines are a certain length and there is no way to increase them, we actually absorb much less.

How do you know if you have an intolerance when you don't know how long it will take for your body to react?

It's very simple! By blood test – f79 Gluten or by biopsy of the small intestine. Of course, crunching chips with Coca Cola or eating another sweet candy, I don't think there is a need for tests. Are you following my thought?

Don't worry! Only 0.3–1% of people suffer from gluten intolerance. But still there is, unfortunately, an increase in this number!

The symptoms by which you can tell that gluten is not for your child are

diarrhea,

bloated belly,

swelling,

irritability or

slow weight gain and development.

Symptoms in adults are

depression and anxiety,

herpes, mouth ulcers (immune system is weak),

fatigue and poor health,

imbalance in hormones,

anemia, muscle or dental problems or

appearance of gas in the stomach.

Always clean the dining and cooking area as well as the dishes! And now let me reassure you that a gluten-free life is not deprivation or suffering.

Gluten-free foods are extremely tasty and varied:

fruits and vegetables,

unprocessed seeds and nuts,

any fresh meat,

fish,

eggs,

amaranth, arrowroot, buckwheat, flax, quinoa, tofu, millet, peas, lentils, beans, chickpeas, einkorn,

potatoes,

rice,

chestnuts and

fresh herbs and spices.

It's not little, is it?

Listen to your body, give it energy and strength!

History is that version of past events that people have decided to accept.

Napoleon Bonaparte I

Dried Fruit – The Illusion

Is it useful or harmful?

Everyone who starts a diet, rushes to replace sweets with dried fruits and honey. Often, even before that we have not even consumed sweets, but from the reduction of food and the wrong combination, the body begins to look for sugars to get the energy it needs.

What is really in dried fruits? There is a very positive charge. Remember the pages I wrote about free radicals and longevity? Well, free radicals shorten it. These are many pluses that are trying to bring down our systems. To stop them, we need minuses.

One fruit has a negative charge, up to 48 hours after it is picked from the tree. We buy the dried fruit long after that. In this way we take many pluses, which we should then neutralize.

When dried, the water and many of the useful properties disappear. The sugars remain.

An apple has 4 tbsp. of sugar. It is glucose and fructose. We have already talked about this. After it dries, both remain. But if it was fresh, you would eat an apple and get full. It has a lot of fiber that would satisfy you and you don't want more. When we make fresh juice or eat dried fruit, we eat only sugar. From the fact that the volume is not there, we can eat a large amount. Which automatically means a lot of sugar. We raise blood sugar and release insulin. It lowers it below normal. And after 20–50 minutes we feel hungry for more sweets.

So, we start eating at intervals of 30 minutes to 2 and a half hours. In one case we raised a lot of blood sugar, and in the other we ate very little protein and fat.

If we have insulin, we gain weight. In the end we are on a diet, we almost don't eat, but we put on weight.

In nature, everything is very cleverly invented. The problem is that as technology advances, we do not eat as nature has intended, but we upset the balance and eat only the part that we have decided is useful. Or just delicious.

Separately, there are fruits that are further processed with sugar to make them sweeter and more desirable. Especially for children. Others are treated with preparations and stabilizers to have a longer shelf life.

The idea is not to replace one sweet with another, but to eat so that you do not feel like eating sweets. If you want sweets, this is most often due to the consumption of light protein or lack of fat in your diet.

The problem is not that you want to eat sweets. The real reason is in your previous meal. That's why I love it when someone tells me "I'm ashamed to write you what I eat." And then I saw candy, dates, dried fruit or coffee. These are the lights that show me where the bug in the system is.

Well, do you eat dried fruit?

Don't answer "rarely." Write down what you eat in 3 days as well as the time. But with an accuracy of a minute and with quantities. Chicken to rice 1:2. And then sit down and read them. You will be surprised how many things you eat without being recorded in your system called the brain. They pass as emigrants who quite well hide their traces in your subconscious.

No wonder. Trust me! Have I ever told you something that doesn't work?

Sit down and write.

Good luck, Fairy!

They say the opposite of noise is silence. That is not true. Silence is merely the absence of noise.

Terry Pratchett

Colic

On 9 June 2018 once again I was lecturing pregnant women and those who gave birth recently, but this time – in Sofia. And I remembered how important the first days of a baby are and how many questions a mother-to-be has.

In the following lines I will tell you things that are valid for both adults and children. The question is to understand my words correctly. Not to read across the lines and say, "I know that!"

First: Many mothers stop breastfeeding because the baby cries, often wakes up in the evening and is hungry. Here I will give you a joker: if you eat more often than 4 hours, your baby will want to eat more often. By "you eat" I mean any salt, nut, candy or coffee that gets in your mouth. Fix your food, start eating right and you won't know you have a baby.

Second: Colic! The horror of a mother. Seeing the little one growl, how his stomach hurts and you can't help him, is a terrible thing. I have experienced it and my hair almost turned white. Until I understood why.

I was told to eat oatmeal with yogurt, butter, chicken. What is happening? Nuts contain inhibitors that are removed after soaking. This is a substance that keeps them from sprouting. The chicken has growth hormones that pass directly into the milk. If we have harmful substances in our cosmetics, many of them pass through the blood into the milk and, also, harass our little one. Dairy products, in turn, have a large amount of casein. In human milk, the casein albumin ratio is 1:1. In all other milks it is 3:1. It's like giving triple coffee to someone who has never drunk coffee! Casein takes 14 days to clear your body. Therefore, if your term is on the thirtieth, then you should stop taking dairy products on tenth. Start breastfeeding. If all is well, eat butter once. See how the baby is.

If the baby is fine, then eat dairy. If he cries, you will need 7 to 14 days to clean up. So, try a little. If you have pimples on your forehead or blackheads on your face, then you do not absorb it yourself!

Gluten is another protein that is difficult for the baby's tummy to digest, but by processing it, the mother makes it much more acceptable in breast milk. If you have a tendency to pigmentation and pimples in the lower part of the jaw, then you do not absorb it 100%. In this case, for your health, I recommend that you remove it from your diet.

Keep in mind that everything you eat raises your blood sugar and raises your baby's blood sugar. And if you're sick of eating pies, think about how much value you give to your child. White flour, white sugar, dairy products cause swelling in the body and brain. You swell the most from the salt. If you feel like eating cheese, olives or something salty, you have a mineral deficiency. These are the building blocks. They are obtained from salt. But only from coarse sea salt. It is gray and greasy. Himalayan is also not good.

If you want yellow cheese, butter, yogurt – you need protein and fat.

Think about what you eat. Don't play with yourself and the little innocent soul who relies on you.

Do you know why many mothers have gained a lot of weight in the last months of pregnancy? From their improper diet. You know, by putting water in a saucepan and pouring oil, how the oil is on top. Well, your belly is the pot. Baby is butter. It cannot come down if it is fat. Then the mother begins to gain weight and internal fat. This applies pressure and pushes the fetus down.

Most People Suffer from Their Expectations Colliding with Reality

What is disappointment? Why do we get disappointed?

Everyone sets goals for themselves. Everyone decides where their bar is. We set our own boundaries. They appear first in our consciousness and then become a projection in our daily lives. It is no coincidence that we have fears. And not by chance, every day someone overcomes his fears.

When we raise the bar very high, it is both a plus and a minus. The plus is that we will grow fast. We will progress light years ahead of others. And we will become better at something every day. Better than yourself yesterday!

But there is also danger. Danger of disappointment. Here comes the disappointment, not because we are not good or it did not work out, but because we expected something. And that is exactly what did not happen. Our expectations have not become a reality. If I organize an event for 500 people and 150 come, I will be disappointed. If I organize an event for 2,000 people and 500 come, I will still be disappointed.

The main problem is that we do not look at what we achieve, but we are always looking for what we do not achieve. From there, our focus shifts. We tune in to do something that actually pulls us back.

And, if you're already wondering what I'm talking about, why are we talking about health issues, I'll explain immediately. You want to lose weight, right? This means losing fat and gaining muscle mass. To raise the energy. To be more productive. And why every time you get on the scales you get angry that you lost only 2 kg in one month? Why aren't you glad that you lost 2 kg in one month. Yesterday Tsveti said, "I was on the beach all morning. I still don't like myself in a swimsuit, I have a lot of flaws!" Believe me, she has no more weight to lose. She has the body of a model for me. And her ass is tighter than girls at the age of 18, But she doesn't like herself yet! And here comes the disappointment.

The very fact that we are disappointed means releasing negative hormones on something that depresses us. Something that changes our focus. Body and mind are frustrated, motivation drops. We hold back again.

If you could reverse the process, would you do it?

It's very simple! Look for something you did well. Look for something you like in yourself! Don't look at the imperfections that are still there. Look how many of them are gone! See how you wear clothes that you haven't been able to wear in years. See how your knee is already visible. And did you notice the change in your mood? And that you are calmer now? Not to mention that you have energy for three! Don't look for wrinkles on your face. Look how the pores have already started to shrink, the color has changed. Wait. One by one!

When you enjoy small successes, you release the hormone of motivation. We have already talked about this. Break the big goals into sub-goals. Don't aim to lose 10 kg, but lose 2 cm. Don't aim to lose weight. Ask to get into clothes you couldn't. Don't just ask for something but ask for it precisely and specifically.

Stop being frustrated, because you will find that whatever you start, you will not succeed. This is how you fall into a cycle of holes and pessimism.

Every night I write a list of things I need to do. For some it is good, for others it is nonsense. For me, it's my way of doing my homework and not wasting time. Every week I set a goal, what to optimize and achieve. All this helps me with the monthly targets I want to achieve. And they lead me to the annuals. And so right on target. And above all, I enjoy the road.

Do not push the breaks yourself. Do not pull back! There are at least four personal consultations every day. And I see the same thing every day. Disappointment. Impossibility to see the achieved results. If you cannot value yourself, no one will value you.

I have 10 years of experience in the field of health. And do you know when customers started trusting me? When I believed in myself!

Believe in yourself! The rest is a matter of time!

You give the meaning of life.

Paulo Coelho

Time here is limited so don't waste it living somebody else's life.

Steve Jobs

How Does the Male and Female Brain Work?

Life is what happens while you are making plans.

John Lennon

Five years ago, a friend of mine, nicknamed Troshana, sent me a video. It was because I kept getting angry at the male audience. And today, unintentionally, I returned to this information. It was insanely useful to me, so I decided to share it with you.

Every single piece of knowledge that makes our life simpler and easier is worth sharing!

Imagine the male brain as a warehouse with thousands of boxes. These big yellow boxes with two holes on the side to lift them. You can't help but see them in the movies, carrying luggage with them. And they are empty. Completely empty. Little by little, over the years, man began to arrange them. Divide them into rooms by theme. Label them in capital letters. But even at the age of 99 there is an empty one in his mind. Even if his place runs out, he will rearrange, make new rooms, throw away old folders and fill the boxes with new ones, but he will not touch this one. It is the way to rest. When he gets tired and his relay overheats, he will sit on the couch, turn on the TV and start flicking through the channels. Or will just stick with one of them. He will start scrolling on his phone. He will do something super pointless, in which he seems to be "wasting his time." And I know that this infuriates us women!!! Ooooh, yes! It can get on our nerves. Especially if we do something and tell him: "Give me this" or "Do this" and he doesn't seem to hear us. It's as if he's disconnected from the world around him. And that's right! He's opened that empty box and his mind is an empty space, without colors and noise, without movement.

I didn't understand this condition before. How the hell are you going to waste your time so aimlessly with a thousand things to do!?! Today I sincerely envy men. This is their way. And it is unique. I can't do it!

But let's see what's going on in a woman's head

Hmmm... it's hard. Imagine neurons. These are nerve cells that look like a dot with many protruding tentacles. These tentacles grasp another neuron. The chain is colossal. Each event catches on to another 10, and some lead to another 1,000. It's like a huge network. Something like the Internet today. Everyone is connected to the other, whether they know it or not. And now imagine how not one impulse walks away in the network, and 20, maybe 50 thoughts are loaded at the same time. This is why women take a break from one activity while doing another. This is not accidental. We were created to be mothers! Only a mother knows what it is like to work, to look after children, a husband and pets. Only she knows how to make sure the child doesn't fall, to iron, to talk on the phone, to listen to the radio to hear what happened, to think about what needs to be done tomorrow and to cook at the same time. I, for example, relax by cleaning. If I'm tired or tense, I lick the entire house clean. Think about it! How do you clean? You go into one room, take toys from the other, laundry from the basket in the hallway and rubber bands from the closet. You take a thrown T-shirt from the cupboard with the keys, go through the other room, then you take a glass of water, some napkins, drop the toys... pass by the kitchen drop the glass, take some rubbish off the floor. In a sense, you don't just clean one thing and do empty courses, but it is as if your terrain is like a map. Every object points to you with an arrow where it is and you just combine the road and the trajectory with it – multitasking.

Hence the various tactics and methods of action in both sexes. Men are one-task. That's why they usually become super good

270

at one thing. And we women are not so good, but we do well in 1,000 things. Here come the disagreements and the scandals. When there is something to be done, we will do it, resting. And the man will sit down and turn himself off. That's why when they say something, they don't hear us.

For us, the only way to drown out the impulses in our consciousness is to hold on and focus on one. Thus, our consciousness rests.

Did you get the difference? I hope you think about it next time before you get angry and release negative hormones.

I don't know what the key to success is but the key to failure is trying to make everybody happy.

Bill Cosby

Thermal or Micellar Water

What is the difference?

A micelle is a small sphere made up of molecules that have a head and a tail (similar to sperm). The round heads are hydrophilic (they connect easily with water), and the tails that remain outside are hydrophobic (they connect with fats). Everyone knows how fat floats above water. This is also the idea behind the mycelium. These little spheres float in the water undisturbed until you put them on a cotton swab.

Cotton, like water, is hydrophilic – that is, the heads are connected to it, and the tails remain outside, lonely, to connect with the oily ingredients on your face – makeup, sebum, impurities. Each tail can bind with a limited amount of fat, so we need to change the cotton particle until we clean the face perfectly. Some people use water for toning as a spray (it is not for that), the face is always wet. Accordingly, mycelium remains on the skin. They bind on the one hand to the skin (water), on the other to sebum and makeup. In this way we make an even stronger connection. Simply put, no one puts soap on their face and goes to bed with it, right? Therefore, always after micellar water, wash your face.

The good thing about micellar waters is that they do not have alcohol or soap, which makes them gentle on the skin.

Thermal water – this is sealed in a package of water from a thermal spring. It should be out of touch with oxygen. Remember the article about free radicals and the negative charge that neutralizes them. The idea here is the same. No free radicals, no aging. At the same time, we absorb much more substances through the skin than through the mouth. Water-thirsty cells absorb like a sponge. Remember the plant you spray to keep it fresh. The purpose of thermal water is to hydrate and soothe the skin, for example, if the baby's bottom is red, if there are irritations, after hair removal to prevent them.

If Somebody Changes, It Is Because They Wanted to and Not Because Somebody Made Them

I don't know if you noticed that I'm not talking about food and exercise. I left the last four chapters to motivate you. I want to give you some examples from life. And make you love what you have. Appreciate it!

When I posted some of my big events and talked about how I was going to change lives, many people responded with the saying, "You can lead a horse to water but you can't make it drink." Many people think they are changing due to external pressure.

Everyone changes because they have decided to. Because they asked for it. The point is that many of us don't know what we can do. What does change mean? What can you change? Today we have so many possibilities that we cannot be born and know them all. Unfortunately, there is no "See what you can do" manual. All books cover specific topics. There is no way to know everything. It is impossible!

After 26 years in sports, food and cosmetics and the knowledge gained from it, I still learn something new every day. As we sleep on the other side of the world, they invent thousands of new things.

I can't make you start eating healthy. Nor can I teach you how to stand upright. If you don't ask. You will ask if you have this need. You've heard of Abraham Maslow's pyramid. And maybe for its modifications. Different needs for security, progress, diversity and fun, significance, love and commitment, contribution to something. Everyone has 6 needs, but at the moment 2 or 3 are dominant. That is why everyone has different needs. For some, health is important, for others, attention and to be attractive, for a third, to go to a disco. Others are on the wave of workaholism – they need security.

That's why people who read my articles and books, watch videos and attend trainings need them. I can't make you buy this book if you don't need it.

The choice is ours. When I met my husband, I fell head over heels in love. I was a bimbo on heels, with makeup, nails, hair extensions, in other words I needed attention! Everyone noticed me. And he asked me to change! To become invisible. He needed security. To know that I will be only with him without danger of anyone taking me away. Sounds like property, but it's true. In finding him, I filled my need for significance. If it hadn't happened, I would never have changed my wardrobe to include sneakers and men's shorts, a white rubber watch and a sports tank top.

We decide for ourselves whether to make a change. If every day someone tells you that you are fat or that you are crooked, if you do not decide to change, it will not happen. You will not come to my training first. Second, you wouldn't buy the book.

That's why there are so many different interests. Some people just want to show off – buy expensive clothes, phones, watches and are happy. Others want to be healthy. They want the certainty that they will live long. Others want to have fun. Find what is important to you. Turn off your conscience! Do not choose security, progress and contribution, because it is fashionable. Choose what is important to you now. And give it to yourself. You will not want to contribute if you are not certain that you will remain healthy. You cannot ask for love from your family if you are a burden to them due to health problems.

You come before everyone!!! You are the most important! If something happens to you, what will the people who love you do? How will you help them if they need you? So don't just read what I'm writing but pull yourself together and do something about it. Set a goal to do something new for you every week.

Something that will help you achieve your goal! Not what people want for you! They don't even know what they want for themselves!

It's very funny to see football fans. You watch an overweight man criticizing a football player about how he failed to score a goal. He describes what he had to do, as if he could do it himself! Well, don't listen to others, listen to what you want! And do it today!!!

You don't need to be great when you start something new but you need to start something new to be great.

Zig Ziglar

It's Never Too Late

Well, we are at the end. Are you ready for me to refute any of your doubts and excuses in your head?

Me – Yes!

Some will say that I will give you only 8 examples. And I will tell you that I will give you the entire 8 examples. Read carefully:

Elizabeth – a 93-year-old lady who can't get up from her chair. But she trains individually with an instructor. He shows her different movements and she applies them sitting in the chair with her legs and arms. The video is astounding, the woman laughs heartily throughout the workout. She shares how she can't wait for the time to train.

Ernestine Shepherd – an 80-year-old bodybuilder. She is officially named the oldest bodybuilder in the world. She started playing sports at the age of 56. She gets up every morning at 2:30 and runs 10 miles. Enters the gym at 4:30 p.m. She then trains from 7 a.m. with a group of people aged 20 to 86. And from 11.30 a.m. she leads a class with 45 people.

Gladys Misiewicz – is 100 years old. She gets up every morning at 4:30 a.m. and participates in all sports activities at Villa Maria in Michigan.

At age 85, Ed Whitlock completed the Toronto Marathon in 3 hours 56 minutes and 34 seconds, becoming the oldest man to run 26.2 miles in less than four hours. He started running at the age of 60.

Sister Madonna Buder, also known as the "Iron Nun," began training triathlon at the age of 48. She participated in her first Ironman at 55 and continues to this day (about 400 triathlons, including 45 Ironman). She has won 11 national titles in the United States, including eight in the Olympic triathlon in the relevant age groups, and is a 1-time world champion with 12 wins in her age group at the Ironman World Championships in Hawaii.

And do you know the story of Stephen King. He was a drunk. He started writing a book, but one day he threw it in the trash. His wife saw it and put it away. They lost everything. They lived in a caravan with their daughter. He would lose them too, but she took out the draft and he completed it. And so, it became the bestseller *It*.

Sylvester Stallone – rejected by his parents due to a disease of the facial nerves and inability to show emotion. Gets married. He has no finances and steals his wife's jewelry. He is left without a roof over his head. He lives alone with his dog in his car. He has no money and sells his dog. Some say it's for $25, others for $100. He's writing a screenplay soon. And he starts looking for a way to sell it. Fails. Receives refusal after refusal. Until one day they say yes to him. They offer him $250,000, but he refuses and says he wants to play the lead role. They offer him $350,000 and only want the script. He refuses again. He wants to play the lead role with his dog. In the end, they give him $35,000 plus what he wants. The first thing he does is buy back his dog. But his new owner wants $10,000. And today this script is known as the movie *Rocky*.

Another story. An old man named Harland Sanders retired at the age of 65. He is left with only a $65 pension and a homemade recipe for cooking chicken in his head. He starts going from restaurant to restaurant, wanting to sell the recipe. For every portion prepared and sold, he wants 5 cents. He gets refusal after refusal a total of 1008. The 1009th respondent agreed. And so, he sold the recipe to 5 restaurants. In 1963, his recipe for delicious chicken was already sold in 600 restaurants, and the Kentucky Fried Chicken chain was gaining in popularity.

So, Fairy, stubbornness is an important quality. You set a goal and you act. Don't put it off until tomorrow, because tomorrow may never come. And to miss seeing what you can achieve because you are afraid is really sad.

Everyone has something to do in this life. It's up to you whether you go across or around. You can do it in one life, or you can be halfway there in 100. All my life I wanted to study rehabilitation, beauty, health, and movement at a sports academy. And all my life someone has been pulling me in another direction. It took me many years to realize it. And every time I started something, sooner or later it took me there again.

When you want something, you can't fool yourself with excuses that something else is better, because... sooner or later it will strike you again. Instead of meandering through the small dark streets, go across and don't be surprised. You know that life is not measured by the number of breaths, but by the moments that take your breath away.

The worst thing that can happen to me is to be like everybody else.

Arnold Schwarzenegger

Focus On: Emiliya Belcheva

Emiliya Belcheva has been an expert in beauty and health for more than 10 years. She is the only international lecturer and coach in FaceBuilding in Bulgaria, and is also the founder of the Belchevi Health Academy. Creator and trainer of SEMMA. She is the only Beauty Coach for Bulgaria. She does all this in order to help everyone who wants to change and become healthier, more beautiful and the best possible version of themselves.

At first glance, my acquaintance with Emiliya Belcheva was accidental, but I haven't believed in coincidences for a long time. Very soon after, I realized that it had appeared in my life at a time when I was ready to perceive everything that spread fascinatingly as knowledge. Her appearance as a girl with natural beauty and a responsive attitude attracts instantly, but the wisdom in her words and her extensive knowledge in the field of health and beauty make her a truly valuable interlocutor with whom time passes imperceptibly fast. I can't hide that it was a real pleasure for me to recharge from her energy and I tried to "absorb" everything I heard while doing this interview. Here is what Emiliya Belcheva shared for the readers of LAZARA.bg:

LZ: What is SEMMA?
SEMMA is a sport that I invented after being injured by all kinds of sports activities that I practiced over the years and after my two births. I had a lot of distortions, varicose veins and damage after pregnancy. I had to stop training, spend many hours in rehabilitation and not have time for my family. That's why I chose to combine corrective gymnastics with spinning and two breathing techniques entered in the Guinness Book of Records. Thus, within 4 hours a week, I cured scoliosis, erased cellulite, removed varicose veins and straightened my posture. I increased my energy, improved my memory and cleared my

skin. My panic attacks are gone. I have genetically encoded diseases, expressed in nervous attacks, panic attacks and suffocation (asthma). With the training, they also disappeared. Due to oxygen saturation and the straightening of the posture, the metabolic age is reduced. For 16 training sessions, 21 years are reduced.

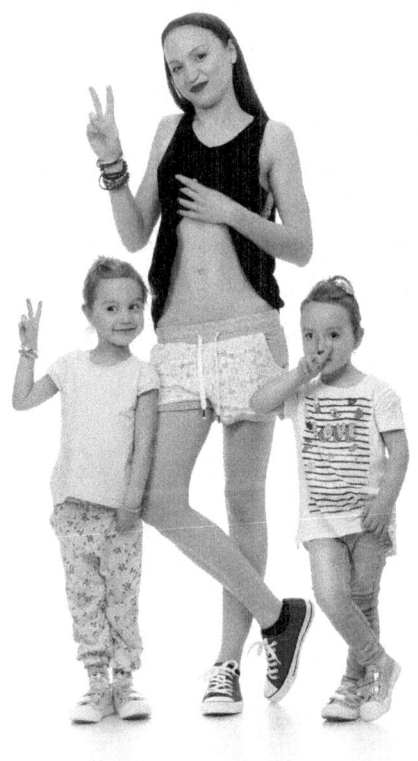

LZ: What is metabolic age?

This is the age at which the tissues and organs in the human body function. For example, I am 30 years old and have two children. My metabolic age is 14 years. Twelve to fourteen years is the minimum for a developed individual. When I train in the country and abroad, it is very frightening when I measure young women at the age of 20 and see that their body age is 53.

The average life expectancy of a woman is 66 years. In reality, their lives are just beginning and their bodies think they are coming to an end.

LZ: What is metabolic age affected by?

By our way of life. This includes when we go to bed, what we eat, what light we stand in, how much and what kind of water we drink, what habits we have, what cosmetics we use (from toothpaste to mascara), ecology and even what kinds of clothes we wear. All this causes the release of stress hormones. Today, the word "stress" is a bit misunderstood. For our body, stress is the artificial substance that touches the skin, the carcinogenic SLS in the toothpaste or in the child's sunscreen, in blue light from the flashing light on the phone by the bed. Stress is also spending a lot of energy on processing food, which does not give us value.

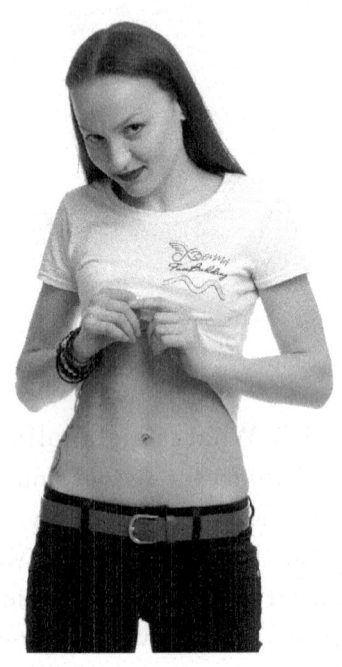

Imagine that the body has 100 units of energy for the day. It is up to us whether we will use them to regenerate the body and prolong life or to fight harmful lifestyles and free radicals. In the first case, we lower the metabolic age, in the second – we increase it. For example, I have trained all my life for a beautiful body and relief from pain. I have always been low in energy and found many shortcomings. Today I train to drop my metabolic age and thanks to that I am focused, I have inexhaustible energy and I really feel like a 14-year-old. Before I trained about 40 hours a week, I had a muffin top and limited my diet. Now I train up to 5 hours a week, I have excluded only three things from my diet and I am in my best shape. I feel perfect. I used to live to train, and now through SEMMA training I change my daily habits to make my life better.

LZ: In recent years the effect of free radicals is very much discussed. Can you say something more about them, different than what we generally hear?

I like to give illustrative examples because it is more understandable and easier to remember. Imagine an inflated balloon with two smaller ones in it. One small bubble is your DNA and the other is your "factory" for energy. There are many sharp pluses between them, which hit everything. Instead of producing energy for regeneration, all resources are redirected to calm the pluses. Regeneration stops. Artificial aging of the cell begins. It is only a matter of time before the pluses crack the DNA wall. Once changed, the body recognizes that it is not its cell. At best, it is destroyed and discarded. At worst, the mutation spreads.

The body has the ability to regenerate itself. We are the ones who hinder it. What neutralizes free radicals is the negative charge. We can get it through raw food. After heat treatment, the negative charge becomes positive.

LZ: How does food affect our mood?

Food determines what hormones are released in our body, and hormones determine what we are. Depending on the metabolic type of a person, one food could have a wonderful effect on one, but an adverse effect on another. For example, if my eldest daughter eats greasy food, she falls asleep, becomes angry and crooked, speaks "in spite" and is irritable. If my little one eats it, she will be productive, smiling, full of energy and concentration.

Many times we have worked with troubled children who are aggressive and have little success in school. With only slight adjustments in the diet, within a month they became smiling and excellent students. And to prove it to you, I'll give you three jokers: if you feel like eating cheese, olives or something salty, then you have a micronutrient deficiency. Start salting with gray, coarse, greasy sea salt. If you feel like eating yellow cheese or need to consume milk, your body lacks fat and protein. And third, if you feel nervous, sad (like most women before their period), eat something fatter and eat more protein, and you will see how you will become the happiest person in the world.

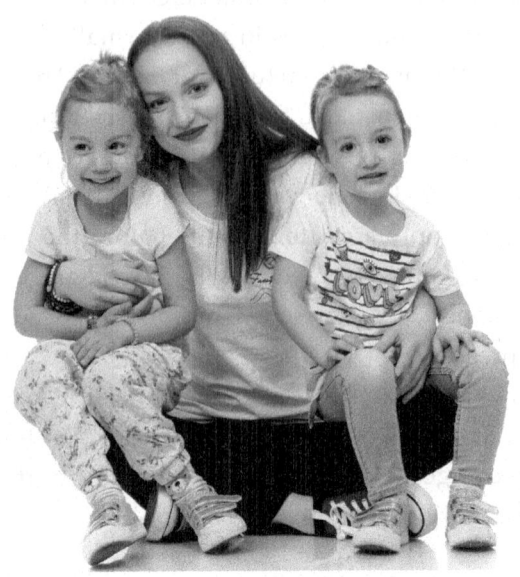

We eat everything for a reason, but because the finished food is too tasty, our receptors are confused. Our skin and emotions show where we are mistaken in our diet.

LZ: You mentioned that you excluded three specific products from your diet. What are they?

These are the three products that cause cellulite, swelling, aging and above all raise the metabolic age. The problem is not that we will wake up with bags under our eyes, but that every time we have them, our whole body, including the brain, swells. The swellings are mainly from white sugar, white salt, dairy products and white flour, but I really replaced the salt with gray coarse and greasy sea salt, not Himalayan. It gives us the necessary trace elements, and the other types of salt extract them. On the other hand, sugar breaks down collagen fibers. This can be seen on the wrinkles on the face. Collagen is our building block, which is in all our tissues, bones and organs. Therefore, wrinkles are our smallest problem, but it is a sufficient indication to understand that we need to do something and prevent things.

It is in order to increase people's knowledge that I started doing Masterclasses and Trainings in different cities. I realized that people have a desire for change, but they don't have the information they need. We look at habits and food as something routine, which does not matter much, but in reality, the quality of our life, how we feel and how we look depends on them.

LZ: I understand that in July you will lower the metabolic age by 20 years of 40 people in 8 days...

You are good! We announced it just 2 weeks ago. Yes, it is correct. I really set a goal to bring 40 people back to life between July 22 and 29. I have invited various mentors from the country and abroad to help me with this. During this retreat, which we called "Raise your quality of life," every day we will have a training in corrective gymnastics SEMMA, one hour of self-massage and one hour of FaceBuilding. The goal is to relax overstretched muscles and tighten atrophied ones. We will check everyone's metabolic types and in 8 days we will make the right combination of foods a habit. We will practice breathing techniques for complete regeneration. The food we will eat is entirely organic and the place we will stay is in the top 10 of *Time* magazine. Exercises and lectures will be practical. Our purpose is not to just drop the metabolic age but build the right habits in those present and teach them how to maintain it.

This has been my dream for 5 years now – to pass on everything I know to many people and, even at the moment, while I am telling you this, I have goosebumps. It is surprising how in just 2 weeks half the seats are already occupied and now I understand that people have a desire for change and this motivates me even more.

And if you're still wondering why I shared it with you? Because it is important to know what you can do! And you decide for yourself if you will do it!

And here I will give you a gift! Take a picture with my book. Send it to my personal e-mail: emiliq.belcheva@gmail.com. I will send you a code and you can use a 15% discount from my books *Regeneration* and *The Bible of a Happy Pregnant Woman*, for a personal consultation or diet. And you can choose a video gift from our site (* massage "Get rid of stress," "Ancient drainage facial massage," "Facebuilding 1,2,3" or "Lifting in 10 minutes").

Life is like riding a bike, we have to move forward so we don't lose our balance.

Albert Einstein

An Inspiring Personal Story

Today I will tell you a personal story about a girl I met recently who inspired me. She inspired me to realize that things we do make a difference even though we don't get the opportunity that often. Words heard in the bus, a sentence read from a book, a smile or a look from a stranger... The exact words in the right moment can change lives. As if we get an enlightenment that others don't see but for us it is like a big road sign that we know is there for us. The personal story shouldn't be masked with pictures and ads so let me just copy the text of the author.

Hi, Ema

just now I see the calendar and on this day a year ago I went to check my tumor markers for my cyst. Nothing is accidental

"Investment in knowledge brings the highest dividends."
Benjamin Franklin

And it is no coincidence that you are reading this!

Hello to all who want to change their lives for the better and to all who are still at a crossroads. GET STARTED!

You will only gain and lose absolutely nothing but your bad habits.

But like most people, as I was, everyone wants to hear from someone what they went through, what happened to them, what changed.

That's why I will tell you my personal story.

To this day, I am a person who does not use anything harmful, or rather those key things. I do not eat ANYTHING WHITE! White flour, white sugar (no sugar), white salt. I also do not eat white rice and dairy products. Many of you will ask yourself, "But I can't, BECAUSE I love cheese, chocolate, white bread." YOU CAN!! I also thought I couldn't, but here I am now. I feel wonderful, energetic, happy, positive.

And what do I look like? First, I will tell you what I looked like before. Because I'm aware that you're tired of reading everywhere, watching videos, dieting and feeling bad, taking vitamins, taking the pills given to you by people in white coats, and getting results in a week or two and then it's all the same again. This demotivates a hell of a lot, you despair, you stop caring about yourself and you say to yourself: "whatever happens, I'm tired, I'm tired of limiting myself and getting no results."

Pimples on the face, missing energy, unradiant skin, breaking hair and nails, too much weight for the wedding in June but in August there is no memory of a diet.

That's why I'm writing these lines, to tell you that there are people who were also like that, they were also desperate, tired of the eternal new and "best thing" and throwing thousands of levs for "top cosmetics" and supplements that "work miracles."

It will be a little longer to read, but I want you to see the whole picture, because everything in this life, in our body and in the universe has a causal relationship. To see the consequences of a little "normal thing".

And I start from the beginning. I was 16 years old, in fact almost 16, it happened 3 days before my 16th birthday. It appeared on my clean face – a large, red and very painful cyst on my left cheek. Now you're going to say to yourself, "Hey, at 16, puberty, that's normal." Yes, but it's not! Of course, the first thing I did was go to a dermatologist. He told me it wasn't acne, it was cysts (because they were starting to come out more). I was given antibiotics and cosmetics to treat externally.

I took the antibiotic for two weeks, did everything as planned, and the situation had improved a little bit. BUT the moment I stopped taking the antibiotic, a week or so later, my face was worse than before. The cysts were already double in size, terribly painful, the moment they burst, there were very deep scars and there you go... this was the beginning of my torment, the end of my clean face.

I have had countless sleepless nights because I was in pain and burning inside. People started telling me: "Stop the chocolate", "Stop the greasy, fried food", "Here's another antibiotic", "Come on, apply it now". And I listened, of course you can't take antibiotics all the time, you need a break and the moment I stopped, the lull was a memory. I went around all the best doctors in dermatology and nothing. There was one left, I went to him, I was already a first-year student at the age of 20, puberty should already be a memory (but not for me). There was always a red and painful bump. I had forgotten that I was very white in general, because my face had always been red for years.

So, I went to the last dermatologist and promised myself: it's over. I listen to what he tells me and I hope it works out. I again gave a solid amount of money for minutes to tell me the following: "Take this pill for a year, during this period you should not get pregnant, every 4 months you should do a full examination of the liver, blood and all the extras. Your hair may start to fall out, your nails may break (in my head was: the end, I have nice nails and thick hair, and somebody tells me to kiss them goodbye), but don't worry the problem will disappear and then everything will come back to normal." I left, I was with my mother, we looked at each other and we just said to ourselves that I would not undergo this, I would go like that, but I would not damage my organs. And so life went on, there was a lull, then they blazed terribly again

289

and so on. While a year ago I had an annual check-up with my gynecologist and he said, "You have a cyst, not a small one on your right ovary, please let us see tumor markers as soon as possible and discuss the options." I was 24 years old, I hadn't given birth. The tumor marker results were not good. The option was surgery, I asked if they gave me a guarantee and they told me "We can't give you a guarantee".

And I said to myself: the end. I talked to my parents and my mother sent me to one of my "Gurus" (I don't mention names, it's too personal!) Things were like this: I change my habits, my food and I am patient or I go, they cut me and it is not clear what will happen.

And I decided, because of all the things I drank, the food I ate, the lifestyle I led, the cyst, the pimples on my face were one part, I started getting a very strong heartbeat, stomach pains every time after eating and swelling. (I want to emphasize that I was not fat, I played sports regularly, BUT life does not like unfinished things, the food was not as it should be and the result was Zero.)

I felt terrible, I was crushed, I was in hospital for a month because I was constantly sick. My body was giving up. I said to myself: there is no time. I decided - I will not have surgery, but the cyst will not stop growing if I do not take measures, the heartbeat will not stop and it will lead to panic attacks. My Guru told me to stop those things and here my journey begins.

I ate sweets, I ate white flour and everything I listed to you, plus more junk food, I smoked cigarettes, and not a few.

I started, changed the food, stopped the coffee (I drank three coffees a day). And I will not lie to you – I had a terrible headache, I was sick the first few days (there is no other way, we poisoned our bodies for years, it is normal). Before I started, like everyone else, I was looking everywhere to read about a person who has been through something like this. At least a little information – but nothing, only the regular ones with excuses and nonsense, which I had seen so much in recent years that I was fed up with, to put it mildly.

And then she appeared: EMA or my other "GURU" AND COMPANION in my way of life. Thanks to my mom, I got to know her work as a start. She showed me a video of her talking about exactly the things I had stopped, I was still abstinent (food is addictive too, mostly harmful, that's why it's produced) and she inspired me not to give up (even she doesn't know it, only you already know it). I still remember the clip, she was with her two princesses and explained how the problem is not in the pimple, not in the wrinkle, but in what is happening inside OUR BODY.

And so, I met her. I tried to understand every single thing and each of them has a lot of logic, but you have to apply them AND HEAR IT, NOT JUST LISTEN TO IT. I finally saw the general idea of the human body, how everything is related to another. Now you're going to say, "Hey, that's clear." It is clear to us, but the goal is to really realize it. When you take action, your body begins to work for you, not against you. Now, if I eat chocolate (I'm still human) then I feel sleepy, I'm nervous, after a few hours I feel like eating again and I have a sour taste in my mouth, then why eat it. As Ema says, "The goal is to hack the system." I came to this conclusion thanks to her.

And I want to insert in capital letters: THIS IS NOT ADVERTISING, THIS IS THANKSGIVING TO HER! I met her from one of her free videos, and they are many, as you know. And she just gave me a really general idea, like I said, there are causal links, and I finally found someone who breaks down from work to explain why and to help us.

But it is all in your hands! So, get rid of your inner resistance, get rid of the excuses: "But I'm at a birthday party tomorrow, so I'll start on another day", "On Monday", etc. Isolate the criticism and resistance of others (they are theirs, not yours!) In the beginning I was hearing a lot of stuff: "You are crazy, eat whatever you want, don't restrict yourself"... today they still find it difficult to start but they say "Wow your face was so bad and now you look so happy" and the like. As grandmas say: "Learn from those who have already been there." So, this is why I share this with you. I started and I inspired my mom, my brother who is 13 years old and now he knows he doesn't need this food. My boyfriend and my dad have big progress, but not like my mother and my brother. But I am patient.

Set a good example, be healthy and inspire your loved ones to be healthy. This is true happiness! Oops and by the way, I promised to tell you how I look now, how I feel and what has changed. My cyst is gone, my facial cysts are gone, my moods, panic attacks and palpitations are gone, my liver is like new, I'm fixing the scars now. I only met Ema this year, even though I've known her for a year and keep an eye on everything she does. She measured my metabolic age and is a 12-year-old girl, unfortunately I had not met her in person before so we can measure my metabolic age before I started, but you can imagine how old the organs have been... I still have a lot to learn, so to you Ema – we will meet often!

Sharing my personal story is an inspiration from my meeting with Emiliya Belcheva! Thank you! Admirations for your work and for your humanity, people like you are rare!

And as I said – start, it's all in the habit and perseverance. Take care of your health, without it everything else loses meaning! I apologize for my mistakes, I'm not a writer, but I wrote it from the heart! Good luck!

E.K.

Twenty years from now you will be more disappointed by the things you didn't do than by the ones you did do. So throw off the bowlines. Sail away from the safe harbor. Catch the trade winds in your sails. Explore. Dream. Discover.

Mark Twain

Smile, Fairy!
The world is waiting for you to enchant it!

We cannot solve our problems with the same thinking we used when we created them.

Albert Einstein

A life-changing book!
Turn routine into something useful for you!

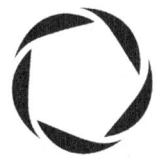

O-BOOKS

SPIRITUALITY

O is a symbol of the world, of oneness and unity; this eye
represents knowledge and insight. We publish titles on general
spirituality and living a spiritual life. We aim to inform and
help you on your own journey in this life.
If you have enjoyed this book, why not tell other readers
by posting a review on your preferred book site?

Recent bestsellers from O-Books are:

Heart of Tantric Sex
Diana Richardson
Revealing Eastern secrets of deep love and
intimacy to Western couples.
Paperback: 978-1-90381-637-0 ebook: 978-1-84694-637-0

Crystal Prescriptions
The A-Z guide to over 1,200 symptoms and their healing crystals
Judy Hall
The first in the popular series of eight books, this handy
little guide is packed as tight as a pill bottle with
crystal remedies for ailments.
Paperback: 978-1-90504-740-6 ebook: 978-1-84694-629-5

Shine On
David Ditchfield and J S Jones
What if the after effects of a near-death experience were
undeniable? What if a person could suddenly produce
high-quality paintings of the afterlife, or if they
acquired the ability to compose classical symphonies?
Meet: David Ditchfield.
Paperback: 978-1-78904-365-5 ebook: 978-1-78904-366-2

The Way of Reiki
The Inner Teachings of Mikao Usui
Frans Stiene
The roadmap for deepening your understanding
of the system of Reiki and rediscovering
your True Self.
Paperback: 978-1-78535-665-0 ebook: 978-1-78535-744-2

You Are Not Your Thoughts
Frances Trussell
The journey to a mindful way of being, for those who want
to truly know the power of mindfulness.
Paperback: 978-1-78535-816-6 ebook: 978-1-78535-817-3

The Mysteries of the Twelfth Astrological House
Fallen Angels
Carmen Turner-Schott, MSW, LISW
Everyone wants to know more about the most misunderstood
house in astrology — the twelfth astrological house.
Paperback: 978-1-78099-343-0 ebook: 978-1-78099-344-7

WhatsApps from Heaven
Louise Hamlin
An account of a bereavement and the extraordinary
signs — including WhatsApps — that a retired
law lecturer received from her deceased husband.
Paperback: 978-1-78904-947-3 ebook: 978-1-78904-948-0

The Holistic Guide to Your Health
& Wellbeing Today
Oliver Rolfe
A holistic guide to improving your complete health,
both inside and out.
Paperback: 978-1-78535-392-5 ebook: 978-1-78535-393-2

Cool Sex
Diana Richardson and Wendy Doeleman
For deeply satisfying sex, the real secret is to reduce the heat,
to cool down. Discover the empowerment and fulfilment
of sex with loving mindfulness.
Paperback: 978-1-78904-351-8 ebook: 978-1-78904-352-5

Creating Real Happiness A to Z
Stephani Grace
Creating Real Happiness A to Z will help you understand
the truth that you are not your ego
(conditioned self).
Paperback: 978-1-78904-951-0 ebook: 978-1-78904-952-7

A Colourful Dose of Optimism
Jules Standish
It's time for us to look on the bright side, by boosting
our mood and lifting our spirit, both in
our interiors, as well as in our closet.
Paperback: 978-1-78904-927-5 ebook: 978-1-78904-928-2

Readers of ebooks can buy or view any of these bestsellers by
clicking on the live link in the title. Most titles are published
in paperback and as an ebook. Paperbacks are available in
traditional bookshops. Both print and ebook formats are
available online.

Find more titles and sign up to our readers' newsletter at
www.o-books.com

Follow O-Books on Facebook at **O-Books**

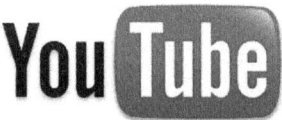

For video content, author interviews and more, please subscribe to our YouTube channel:

O-BOOKS Presents

Follow us on social media for book news, promotions and more:

Facebook: O-Books

Instagram: @o_books_mbs

X: @obooks

Tik Tok: @ObooksMBS

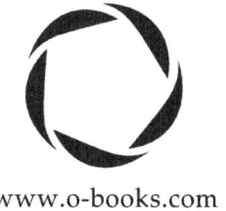

www.o-books.com